Bald
Is Not
an Option

Bald Is Not an Option

Conquering Cancer with Faith, Family, and Your Funny Bone

To Deirdre —
Hang in there!
Love
Tonya Reid
Proverbs
17:22

Tonya Reid

TATE PUBLISHING
AND ENTERPRISES, LLC

Published by Tate Publishing & Enterprises, LLC
127 E. Trade Center Terrace | Mustang, Oklahoma 73064 USA
1.888.361.9473 | www.tatepublishing.com

Tate Publishing is committed to excellence in the publishing industry. The company reflects the philosophy established by the founders, based on Psalm 68:11,
"The Lord gave the word and great was the company of those who published it."

Book design copyright © 2014 by Tate Publishing, LLC. All rights reserved.
Cover design by Joseph Emnace
Interior design by Jomar Ouano
Author Photo credit: Holly Pruitt Photography

Published in the United States of America

ISBN: 978-1-63122-781-3
1. Biography & Autobiography / Personal Memoirs
2. Humor / Form / Anecdotes & Quotations
14.07.23

To Tim, Claudia, and Rachel,
sorry I had to drag you along with me,
but thanks for hanging on all the way.
I love you!

Contents

Part I

My Story

The Wild Ride Begins

I guess I should have seen it coming. I think God gave me a few hints along the way; however, we rarely connect the dots so easily, do we? Two things occurred that, looking back now, I see as God preparing me for my cancer diagnosis. First, I ran across this quote somewhere right before I got the news, and it hit me like a bright red ketchup stain on a new pair of white pants: "When something bad happens, you have three choices. You can either let it define you, let it destroy you, or you can let it strengthen you." Wow! How inspiring. Quotes have always meant a lot to me. I like reading them, passing them along, and applying them to my own life when appropriate. But this quote, I remember reading it and thinking, *Geez, if only people would react like that to life-changing experiences.* Yeah, well, that is very easy to say when it is other people you are talking about, but when you are the one having to decide how to react to a situation, that changes things totally…doesn't it?

The second event that occurred was during the early days of my family's coming to terms with my daddy's cancer diagnosis. Yes, you read it right, my daddy and I both had cancer at the same time! Anyhow, before my diagnosis, I remember having a conversation with my mother about my daddy's cancer and about how his type of cancer was treated successfully all the time now. I vividly remember making these comments, "It's like breast cancer. It's no longer a death sentence. You get diagnosed, treated, and then go on with your life." Again, that is if you're talking about someone else, right…not yourself? Besides, cancer couldn't happen to two members of our family at the same time. That is just against the rules of cancer, isn't it? Oh wait, cancer doesn't play by the rules, does it?

But, friends, that is just what happened. As my precious daddy was making decisions about treatment, choosing doctors, and deciding how to deal with his cancer, the terrible disease made its appearance in my life. It was bad enough that I was having had to deal with it attacking my daddy but to now have to face it head on. I had a husband and two children to think about. I didn't have time for cancer to be rearing its ugly head in my life now. Maybe later, when I was older… much older. Heck, I was only forty-two years old. And I didn't even feel forty-two. Well yeah, when I looked in the mirror, I would see forty-two sometimes, especially if I had waited too long between dye-jobs, but I didn't feel like a grown up. Or sometimes, I would think I was having a conversation with my mother and then suddenly realize that I was just looking in the mirror putting on lipstick. That is how mature I felt most of the time. How was I supposed to make decisions about doctors, treatments, and medications? I could not even make decisions about what to pack in school lunches or whether to go with Tide or Gain when it came to the laundry detergent debate. I still didn't know how to fold fitted sheets for crying out loud. People who have to make decisions about how to deal with cancer should at least know how to fold fitted sheets and have their linen closets in order, right?

But making decisions is exactly what I had to do, and quickly, there was no time to waste. You don't get an instruction manual along with the cancer diagnosis. My husband, Tim, and I learned that you have to maneuver the waters cautiously. We soon discovered everyone has an opinion and likes to tell you what you should and should not do. The type of advice espoused runs the gamut from what doctors to consult, to what foods to eat, and every activity in between. You just have to realize that the people giving this advice love you and really do have your best interests at heart, but you also have to realize that you cannot listen to everyone. God put some very key people in place to guide us though the labyrinth of decision making.

One of the very first decisions that Tim and I made was about the attitude with which we were going to face this health crisis. We had two daughters—Claudia, thirteen years old; and Rachel, eight years old—to think about, and we did not want to be moping around—for God only knew how long—while we dealt with this situation. We didn't want to minimize the seriousness of what was happening, but we also did not want to be overly dramatic—a trait that my family tends to lean toward. We are blessed with fabulous females in our family, which always means we have drama to spare. But in this instance, we were determined that we were going to handle things differently. We were going to stay positive from the get-go and retain our sense of humor through the entire journey. I immediately took Proverbs 17:21–23 as my verse to hang on to through this difficult time. "A cheerful heart is good medicine, but a crushed spirit dries up the bones" (Proverbs 17:22). Maybe it was from desperation or naiveté, but this was the first big decision that we made, and it really did make all the difference in the days that followed.

The first part of my book tells my story. I will admit that exaggerations and embellishments have been made for the sake of a good laugh. Those of you facing your own battle with cancer will identify with many of the issues and circumstances in this part and will realize that you have to laugh in order to avoid tears during many of the situations with which you are bombarded. I hope that by relating my journey, I am able to give hope, compassion, or just a laugh or two along the way. It really is possible to fight this thing with a funny bone. Even though there are plenty of tears as you trudge along, there can be just as much, or more, laughter. The second part of my book relates some lessons or truths that I have come to appreciate through my battle with cancer. I mentioned my affinity for quotes. Early in my journey, my mother began the practice of texting me a TOD (thought of the day) each morning. I have used some of my favorites at the beginning of each chapter. I hope and pray that something in these pages will help those dealing with cancer extract something from my story that might help you deal with what you are facing, even if it is just a chuckle or two; and if that chuckle can get your mind off of your troubles for even just a second, all of this hard work will have been worth it.

Seek and Ye Shall Find

If you aren't in over your head, how do you know how tall you are?

—T. S. Eliot

On a quiet August night, as I was sitting in bed reading *Mudwoman* by Joyce Carol Oates (which, by the way, is the story of a woman who, at a young age, was thrown in a mud pit and goes on to slowly lose her grip on reality...foreshadowing much?), I reached across the bed to grab the remote control (yes, I can multi-task). That is when I first felt something odd. When I investigated further, I realized that there was, in fact, a lump on my left breast that should not be there. I did not immediately panic...much. I simply jumped out of bed, ran frantically into the living room, and tried to form a comprehensible sentence to explain to my husband why I needed to check on our burial policy at eleven thirty at night. He finally calmed me down after my much crying, wailing, and gnashing of teeth. Frankly, I think I just wore myself out. We finally rationally discussed this *thing*. He convinced me it was nothing. It had to be a fibroid cyst. I had no history of breast cancer in my family. It couldn't be anything to worry about. Tim had done a good job of lulling me into a relative sense of peace. Actually, by that time it was probably 1:00 a.m., so I probably passed out from exhaustion.

I called my doctor's office first thing next morning, and my OB/GYN worked me in immediately. This was our first miracle since it normally takes a year to get an appointment. When my doctor examined me, she thought the lump felt like a fibroid cyst. She tried to aspirate it in the office but was unable to do so. I am not sure of the correct medical definition of aspirate. All I know is that it involved a big needle being stuck straight into the worrisome lump. I remember the conversation going something like this: "Okay, Tonya, I am going to ever so gently insert this 30-foot needle into your delicate breast, and the lump will be quickly aspirated, and you can go on with your day with no more worries," said Dr. Snowden.

"Sure," I replied through my sobs.

"This should just take a minute," Dr. Snowden went on as she began the process. "Oh dear, hmmm. This isn't responding the way I thought it would."

"Waaaaaaaaaaa," I screamed. "Maybe you should try a 40-foot needle."

"Now calm down. Just because I can't take care of this in the office, doesn't mean we need to worry yet."

"Of course it doesn't. Excuse me a minute while I call to make an appointment with a lawyer to draw up a will. Do you think if I can't see a lawyer today, tomorrow will be too late?"

"Now don't be a drama queen!" Dr. Snowden scolded. "We just need to get you an appointment for an ultrasound and a mammogram to see what is going on. Let's not get overly concerned yet."

"No, of course not," I promised. "I almost never let my mind run away with morbid thoughts of terrible things that could but probably will never happen to me. I'm good." Dr. Snowden patted me on the shoulder and assured me things would be okay. Arrangements were made for me to travel to Birmingham, the big city about sixty miles away, for the next tests, and I was sent on my way.

I headed home in a sort of fog. I could not comprehend that I may actually have cancer; yet, I knew that I had that lump in my breast. Why, oh why did I have to find that stupid lump? I can't ever find anything. I hide Christmas gifts in places so my children won't find them, and then I am the one who never finds them. I can't tell you the number of times my younger daughter, Rachel, found a wrapped Christmas gift in July stashed behind the piano and wanted to know why Santa didn't put it under the tree. We don't have a key to our house because I have lost so many of them. If our garage door opener ever stops working, so we can enter the house through the garage, we will be homeless. I can't find my sunglasses, I can't find my grey tennis shoes that I have worn exactly two times, and I can't find my tweezers. I can never find a thermometer when one of my girls may have a fever. If we ever need to wrap a gift, I just have to go buy new Scotch tape because I certainly can't find any at home…yet I can find a lump buried deep in my breast. How wild is that. All I kept thinking was that God must have wanted me to find it for a reason because he certainly doesn't want me to find my sunglasses, or he wouldn't keep hiding them from me.

Going Through the Motions

The only way to make sense out of change is to plunge into it, move with it, and join the dance.

—Alan Watts

The ultrasound and mammogram were relatively uneventful. After these procedures, I was told to go home and wait for the results. I remember that a few days passed with no word. I was still holding out hope that all of this was going to end up with the words "fibroid cyst" and "absolutely no reason to worry," and I would quickly forget about this entire incident. Instead, I checked the mail. It was a Friday afternoon after lunch when I got the letter that said something to the effect that my mammogram and ultrasound had shown irregularities. I was urged to contact a surgeon immediately to discuss the next step in my treatment plan, and I had to sign a form and mail it back as proof that I had received this information. Now I was getting worried. A lot worried. I didn't even realize that I had a treatment plan, and the only surgeon I knew was the ENT who had taken out my daughter's adenoids a few years earlier. Pretty sure he didn't want to get my call, so I frantically called my OB/GYN's office. It took about five minutes for the nurse to be able to understand through my sobs what I was talking about. She was very kind and finally gave me the names of two surgeons at St. Vincent's Hospital in Birmingham; however, she gingerly cautioned me that it was a Friday afternoon, so she didn't know if either office would be opened. I took the names and numbers and started dialing.

I didn't get an answer at the first office I called, so I tried the second. Finally, I got an answer. I explained my situation and made an appointment for the following week. Things were starting to get strange at this point. Too much was occurring too fast. I began to feel as if I were existing in an alternate universe. This could not be happening to me. This was not in my plan. I should be running marathons, doing mission work, keeping my house spotless and in order, cooking gourmet meals… oh, maybe that was the alternate universe. Up to this point, only a few close friends knew about what was going on. I had shared the situation with my sister, Aundrea, but had not yet told my parents. I was trying to wait until I had to tell them. Tim and I were trying to keep things as normal as we could for the girls and not alarm them at this point. Turns out, we would have to share all of the details with them soon enough. I went to the appointment at the surgeon's office. Apparently, there was not only the lump I felt on my left breast but another suspicious place on my right breast of which I had not been aware. The surgeon wanted to go ahead and do a biopsy on the place on my left breast in her office the day of the appointment. It was unpleasant but not unbearable. She was unable to do the biopsy on the right breast in the office because of the location of the spot. I would be required to have a biopsy guided by an ultrasound for that breast. She made an appointment for me for this procedure. She told me that she would call me one or two days after the ultrasound procedure with the results.

This is the point in the story when things really begin to get crazy. As I mentioned earlier, my dad had been diagnosed with cancer just a few short weeks earlier before I began my foray into all things malignant. Would you believe that the day that my dad was scheduled for surgery was the same day that I was scheduled to have my ultrasound procedure? I cannot make stuff like this up. Same hospital. One hour apart. I do not kid. Now since my parents did not even know that I had discovered a suspicious place or that anything was amiss, it was going to be hard to explain why I would be running out the day of my daddy's surgery for a procedure at the hospital. My mother tends to be high-strung, some may say neurotic, when dealing with tense situations, so I knew she would not take it well for me to disappear for a few hours on the day of my daddy's *cancer* surgery. My sister begged me not to tell mother and daddy about what was going on. She was convinced it would send them right over the edge. She promised that she would cover for me at the hospital on the day of the surgery by telling mother that I had stepped out to the cafeteria when I needed to make my exit for my appointment. I told her I did possess a healthy appetite, but that even I didn't think Mother would believe I could stay gone wolfing down barbeque sandwiches and key lime pie for two and a half hours. All I could imagine was a "Who's On First" scenario:

MOM: Where's Tonya?

AUNDREA: Who?

MOM: Tonya, your sister.

AUNDREA: Oh, maybe she went to the restroom.

MOM: No, I was just in there. She's not there.

AUNDREA: Who?

MOM: Tonya, your sister.

AUNDREA: Oh, well, maybe she ran to the cafeteria.

MOM: Why don't you go check and see if she's there?

AUNDREA: Where?

MOM: The cafeteria.

AUNDREA: Oh, are you hungry? What can I go get for you?

MOM: No I'm not hungry! I'm looking for Tonya.

AUNDREA: Who?

MOM: Tonya. I'm looking for Tonya! You said she may be in the cafeteria.

AUNDREA: Did she go eat and not ask if we wanted anything? How rude!

MOM: I don't know. I just want to know where she is.

AUNDREA: Who?

Yes, I can just imagine how that would have gone over. I just could not bring myself to keep it from them, so I decided to tell Mother and Daddy about my impending procedure and about all that had been going on. I drove to their house and spilled the beans. I was careful to present everything in the best possible way that I could, still believing that it was a fibroid cyst that I was dealing with. I must say, they took the news much better than I expected. I had underestimated their ability to keep their wits about them. It is not the first time I have underestimated my parents and their ability to love and accept what they must. I am sure they held it together for my sake only. They reassured me, affirming what I already believed, that we had no history of breast cancer in my family but recounting just how many of our women had dealt with fibroid cysts. At least now I would not have to play 007 on the day of Daddy's surgery.

This Is Not a Good Time for Me. Cancer, Can We Reschedule?

Believe you can and you're halfway there.
—Theodore Roosevelt

The day of Daddy's surgery finally arrived. Mother was a nervous wreck, just as we expected. A waiting room full of people spent the day keeping her occupied. I discreetly slipped out, had my procedure done, and slipped back in. The doctor who performed the needle biopsy looked to be about twelve years old and felt the need to explain every movement and action that she was executing during the course of the procedure. She would not be deterred from her explanations by my closed eyes, clenched teeth, and balled up fists as she worked. "I am now getting the needle ready to insert. I am now moving the needle toward your breast. I am now preparing to insert the needle into your breast. I am now going to push down to biopsy the tissue…" said Dr. Twelve Years Old. This was too much information for me. I just wanted her to be finished already! Gotta give the doctor props for being thorough, even if I just wanted her to be through!

The gauze and surgical tape sticking out of the top of my shirt when I returned to wait on Daddy were the only evidence that anything unusual had gone on, well that and my pallid complexion. Daddy came through his surgery with flying colors. The first thing he wanted to know when he woke up from anesthesia was how I was. Oh, how I love my daddy! Now, all I had to do was wait to hear from my doctor. I was feeling pretty good about things. Daddy had done well in his surgery. His doctor felt like he had gotten all of the cancer during surgery, and no other treatment would be necessary. Hallelujah! We were celebrating this news. I was busy convincing myself that my news would be good too. School was starting in a few days. We were busy buying school supplies, going shopping, and looking forward to a new school year.

The surgeon had told me that it may be one or two days before she got the results back. So I waited. I finally got the call on a late Tuesday afternoon. She did not give me the news I had convinced myself I would receive. She said I had breast cancer. What? More specifically Invasive Ductal Carcinoma. Wait a minute…this could not be right. Maybe Dr. Twelve Years Old had made a mistake. Could that be possible? No? I could hardly believe it. I had no family history of breast cancer. I was only forty-two years old. The school year was just beginning. My girls were involved in so many activities at the time. It was just not a good time for me. Couldn't cancer wait? I just didn't see how

I could work it into my busy schedule at the moment. Let's see, Rachel had gymnastics on Mondays and piano on Tuesdays. Claudia had band practice after school on Mondays, Tuesdays, and Thursdays. We had church on Wednesday nights and football games on Friday nights. We had church on Sundays. Okay, so I could possibly do cancer on Saturdays when we didn't have band competitions or birthday parties. I could barely pencil in enough time do laundry, so my family could have clean undies to wear every day. I just did not see how this would work out at all. I need time to plan. I am not a spontaneous kind of person. How can this just be thrown at me with no warning? This was not good, not good at all. I needed some kind of outline or calendar, so I could integrate cancer into my schedule. Wasn't there some kind of *Cancer How To* book out there?

Unfortunately there was not. It seems as if cancer affects each person differently. Stupid cancer! This just keeps getting worse and worse. I hate not being able to control what is happening in my life. Hmmm. Maybe that is what God is planning on teaching me through this whole process...that I am not in control. If that is what he has up his sleeve, I sure hope he sends me an itinerary.

Do We Get a Family Discount?

A happy family is but an earlier heaven.

—George Bernard Shaw

I cried. I prayed. I mourned. I told my family and close friends. Once again, I had to make a visit to my parents' house. My dad had left surgery with the belief that all of his cancer had been removed, and he would probably need no other treatment. However, on his follow-up visit after surgery, his doctor gave him the news there was some evidence his cancer had spread outside of the area removed. His doctor now recommended he go through radiation treatment. Since the day of my daddy's surgery, all my parents had been waiting on was the official all-clear from daddy's doctor, so they could make reservations at the beach and start enjoying a long overdue vacation. Now, with this news, they would have to put those plans on hold to plan Daddy's radiation treatment. He and my mother had just gotten home from the visit where they received this news when I knocked on their door. We exchanged hugs and tears and were having a conversation about

Daddy's situation. They had been on an emotional roller coaster that day, and they were in a very fragile state of mind, so I was very careful to wait for the perfect, ideal moment to bring up my news.

"So I will take the radiation treatments, and the doctor thinks that will take care of everything. Not the news we wanted to get, but we will take it day by day, and we'll get through this," Daddy explained stoically.

"Dr. Tully wants to be one hundred percent sure that there are no more cancer cells, and he says radiation is the way to ensure that," Mother stated as she fought back tears.

Daddy continued, "I have decided to take the treatment in Birmingham. It will probably be five days a week for seven weeks. I know that is a long…"

"I have breast cancer," I suddenly blurted out.

Silence. Mother and Daddy looked at one another, puzzled. It is as if time stopped for a moment.

"W-W-What?" Mother finally sputtered.

"I have breast cancer." I said again. This time they may have actually been able to understand me. Maybe not the perfect moment to break the news but at least I had it out there now.

Both of my parents got up and walked over to where I was sitting and wrapped their arms around me. Hug. I may have been forty-two years old, but I still wanted my Mother and Daddy when I was sick. Perfect. We cried and talked, and I told them the whole story. I could not have asked for more supportive parents. Even in the midst of their turmoil, they were there for me one hundred percent. I should not have expected any less of them. They have always been the parents everyone wished they had. If I had decided to become a tattoo artist, they would have been first in line to have one of my masterpieces inked on their biceps. They are just that kind of people. They have always been right there when I needed them. And boy did I need them now!

Oh, how I wish it were different, and I could be the one to offer the support through Daddy's time of need. It just wasn't in the cards though. We would all have to be there for each other during the coming months. It may get harried and confusing with appointments here and treatments there, but I had a feeling we would make it work somehow. We always seemed to. I just wish we could have gotten some kind of family discount or group rate for having to go through cancer at the same time. It would have been nice to have gotten a discount gas card because we both had to make so many trips back and forth to the doctor or maybe free parking in the hospital parking garage since two family members were members of The Cancer Club. Unfortunately, no one ever offered us these perks, and we just fumbled our way through our situations the best we knew how.

The Right Guy for the Job

That bump in the road you just hit used to be a
mountain, but God got to it first and knocked
it down for you.

—Elmer Laydon, *The Whisper of God*

Now Tim and I had to start making some big
decisions. One of the most important decisions
we made was to get a second opinion. After seeking
advice from several sources, we were led to Dr. Phillip
Fischer. Dr. Fischer is a young doctor. He is probably
around my age, and I definitely consider that to be
young. He is soft spoken, and he looks you in the eye
when he is talking to you. He explains things but not
to the mind-numbing degree of Dr. Twelve Years Old.
I think he can sense just how much a patient can take.
He drew me a picture, yes, drew me a picture, and I
went back to that picture many times after that initial
appointment. Dr. Fischer looked over all of my test
results. He talked with us and explained that I would
need surgery to remove the tumor. He went through
all of the possibilities, explaining about recurrence

rates and such. He told us all about lumpectomies, mastectomies, and bilateral mastectomies. He told me stuff that I thought I would never have to listen to. He also said that after surgery, I would more than likely need chemotherapy and probably radiation because of the size of my tumor.

Dr. Fischer wanted me to have a PET scan to make sure the cancer had not spread to any other parts of my body. Hmmm…hadn't even considered that. Something new to worry about now. Again, ignorance is bliss. Dr. Fischer sent his nurse in to make the arrangements for the PET scan. At this point, the nurse did something that really took us by surprise. She prayed with us. Yes, that is right, she prayed with us. She prayed for peace, for healing, for discernment in decision making. Oh, how I wish I could remember every word of her sweet prayer, but it really doesn't matter. All that really mattered at that moment was that she prayed. That she asked The Great Physician to take care of me and my family. That was when I knew we were in the right hands. This was probably the first time that we had felt peace since I had found the awful lump.

I had the PET scan, and we anxiously awaited the results. Dr. Fischer called a few days later with the news we wanted to hear. The cancer was contained to the left breast. Praise God! I had a follow-up appointment with Dr. Fischer a few days later to move the process along. A very good friend of mine, Ashley Crowson, who also happens to be a nurse, showed up unexpectedly at this appointment to be with Tim and me. She earned the nickname "The Stalker" because she was always popping up when I least expected her (and most needed her). At this appointment, Dr. Fischer talked to us more about what to expect from surgery. I had made up my mind that I would have a double mastectomy. Dr. Fischer had told me at my last appointment the recurrence rate in the unaffected breast is about one percent per year after cancer is removed from the affected breast. Since I was only forty-two years old, I had a great chance of recurrence if I chose a lumpectomy or the removal of only one breast. I just could not imagine ever having to go through all of this again. What if cancer reared its ugly head again when one of my girls was planning a wedding or having one of my grandchildren? No way, that was something I just could not deal with. Getting rid of both breasts was really a no-brainer for me. The sooner the better!

I know for some women, the idea of a double mastectomy is unthinkable. That was not the case for me. I have always cared about my appearance, but the idea of a mastectomy didn't frighten me. I guess I should say the idea of a mastectomy didn't frighten me as much as the idea of death from breast cancer frightened me. Yes, that is more like it. Of course I was worried about the surgery, recovery time, and life after, but I just wanted to get on with the process, so I could get on with my life. I did not like this business of constant doctors' appointments and tests. I had stuffed by bra before, and if need be, I could stuff my bra again. I just wanted to get back to some kind of regular routine that was not interrupted by trips to Birmingham, calls to the doctor, and constant worry.

Let me get back to my daily life of dirty clothes, trips to Wal-Mart, and dinners from McDonald's. Oh, how heavenly that sounded. Maybe God wanted me to learn to be content in my own circumstances through this pilgrimage through cancer. Hmm…possibly. Well, at least we knew we had found the right doctor to lead the way.

I'll Never Be a Barbie Doll

> You grow up the day you have your first real
> laugh—at yourself.
>
> —Ethel Barrymore

D r. Fischer soon asked me a question that I had not even thought about up to this point. He asked me which plastic surgeon I wanted to use. Well, that was like asking me what I was going to say when I accepted my Nobel Peace Prize. The answer to both questions—I don't know. I didn't think I would ever in my wildest dreams have to worry about either one, so I had never given any thought to either. Luckily, Ashley (aka "The Stalker") was at the appointment with me when Dr. Fischer asked this very important question. She was in "the know" about all things medical and was able to offer some guidance on this subject. One of the plastic surgeons Ashley suggested was located right down the hall from Dr. Fischer's office. Dr. Fischer said he worked with this plastic surgeon quite often and felt very comfortable with his work. Convenience and an affirmative nod from Dr. Fischer…Sold! That is how Dr. Michael Beckenstein became my plastic surgeon.

Dr. Fischer's sweet nurse, Teresa, said she would call and make me an appointment with Dr. Beckenstein. She left the three of us, Tim, Ashley, and me, in the exam room. She came back a few minutes later and told us she had called Dr. Beckenstein's office, and that he could work me in right now for a consultation if I wanted to go ahead and see him. If I wanted to? Of course I wanted to! This would save us from having to drive back to Birmingham for yet another day for yet another appointment. Tim and I were beginning to feel like we were living the movie *Groundhog Day*. We would wake up each day, drive to St. Vincent's Hospital to see some doctor or have some test, drive home, go to bed, and wake up to do it again the next day. Being able to see Dr. Beckenstein like this was amazing, but something even more incredible happened next.

Ashley, Tim, and I made our way down the hall to Dr. Beckenstein's office. I so did not want to go in the door. All I could imagine were plastic Barbie dolls excited for their breast enhancements sitting in the waiting room. And even though I would love to be, I faced the truth a long time ago—I will never be a Barbie doll. That required too much work like diet, exercise, and surgery, oh my! People would think I was there for a boob job. Well, I was, but not that kind…not because I wanted to. I didn't choose to be here. I was so embarrassed to go in. I was letting my pride get the best of me. This is where God gave me a huge surprise. We all walked through Dr. Beckenstein's office door. I was shuffling in, looking at the floor, so no one would recognize me and dare think I was there for elective breast enhancement. I finally worked up enough courage to slowly raise my head and look around the room. That was when I recognized a familiar face. It was the face of a lady that I had met through my job, Carol Harcrow, and I knew she had recently been diagnosed with breast cancer. She said, "Tonya, what are you doing here?"

I met her eyes and choked out, "Carol, it's not good." She walked over and hugged me and cried with me. If that is not a God thing, I don't know what is. Carol and I talked. My husband talked to Carol's husband. Ashley talked to everyone. Carol was just a little ahead of me in the process. She had already had surgery and started chemotherapy. She gave me a card from the place where she got her wig. She held my hand. She gave me advice. She told me it would be okay. She will never know just how much her mere presence in that doctor's office meant to me at that moment.

Finally, the nurse called us back. First, we had to watch a video. I think it showed the different options for breast implants. Mostly, we giggled through the whole thing. Ashley was very good at comic relief, so that was another good thing about having her around that day. She never let us get too down. She always found a way to lighten the mood. Finally, I met with Dr. Beckenstein. He explained all of the options for breast reconstruction. One option included a tummy tuck. Somehow the excess tummy skin is pulled up and used in the reconstruction process. This sounded great until I learned that it extended the recovery time. Not for me. I certainly had excess tummy skin that could be used, but I wanted my recovery to be over yesterday. As enticing as a tummy tuck sounded, I would have to pass on it. I certainly was not voluntarily signing up for anything that was going to cause me any excess pain or difficulty. I am all about comfort and convenience. Finally it came time for the examination.

I guess I thought by this time all of the embarrassment of exposing myself would have been gone since I had been stripping pretty much daily for a variety of doctors, nurses, technicians, and various hospital employees. At one point, Tim and I stopped in at the hospital coffee shop. The little guy who was working mistakenly put whipped topping on Tim's cappuccino. When Tim asked him to "take it off," I started coming out of my shirt right in the middle of Starbucks! I started thinking my parents had wasted their money on my college education since it appeared that stripping had become my daily practice.

Dr. Beckenstein explained he would follow Dr. Fischer in the operating room on the day of surgery. Dr. Fischer would perform the bilateral mastectomy, and then Dr. Beckenstein would start the reconstruction process. He would insert tissue expanders at that point. The easiest way I can explain about tissue expanders is to compare them to water balloons. They are deflated when inserted, and then I would have to go to Dr. Beckenstein's office once a week after surgery to have the expanders "pumped up" with a saline solution. This stretches the skin in preparation for the final breast implants after all treatments such as chemotherapy and radiation. I was so glad to find out the expanders could be put in when the breasts came off, like all mothers know… you can't pass up a good BOGO deal.

Now let me just say I was extremely thankful for what Dr. Beckenstein was going to be able to do for me. I realized that reconstruction was a luxury many women who have traveled this road in the past did not have available to them. I also realized that eventually, Dr. Beckenstein would probably work his magic and make me look even better down the road than I did at that very moment. Having said all of that, I think I would have rather faced a clique of gum-chewing teenage girls while wearing a pair of mom-jeans and the wrong shade of lipstick than to have faced an appointment with Dr. Beckenstein. The encounter with the girls would probably wreck my self-esteem less than seeing a plastic surgeon. Let me explain for those of you who don't happen to have your own personal plastic surgeon like I do.

Apparently, plastic surgeons love mirrors. I don't really understand this, but most patients must really enjoy admiring themselves in the mirror while the doctor is doing his examination. Of course, all the mirrors did to me was send me in to involuntary spasms. I was so busy jerking my head from left to right in an effort to avoid having to look directly in the mirror at myself during the awful examination that I'm surprised I didn't come out of there in a neck brace. Then, there was always a nurse in the room too, so that made it extra awkward for all of those in attendance. That day, after

I had been through about a half a box of tissue while whipping my head back and forth trying not to catch a glimpse of anything, I guess the nurse felt like she needed to console me some. She stayed and talked to me as I cried. I think the nurse must be a nurse, hippie, or poet. She proceeded to tell me that God uses strong women for warriors, and I will fight my way through this. She said that when I am on the other side of this, I will be a mentor for someone just as someone will walk me through. Then she said something about teardrops being like rain and washing away the dust...I didn't get that part, but I loved the part about the warrior woman! I thought I would hold on to that. Tonya, the Warrior Woman. Look out, Katniss! I liked that a lot better than Barbie.

That Which Does Not Kill You, Probably Gives You a Migraine

You never know how strong you are until being strong is the only choice you have.

—Cayla Mills

We scheduled a date for the surgery, and I started to get myself prepared. Of course getting prepared included shopping! My mother, sister, and I went on a shopping spree for post mastectomy essentials. What did that include, you may ask? Well, I didn't know, but I will use any excuse to go shopping. I chose new pajamas, which buttoned up the front. We all assumed those would be needed. I purchased a new robe and slippers for the hospital stay. Hey, no need to look lousy just because I may feel lousy for a while. I am a big believer in the old saying, "If you look good, then you feel good." I probably would not feel good for awhile after my surgery, but I figured that new, cute pajamas would certainly help, at least a little.

The day for surgery arrived. Tim, my girls, and my parents arrived at the hospital at the crack of dawn, as instructed, to wait for hours until I was taken back for surgery. Isn't that the way it always works? Before surgery, I was taken for a lovely little procedure called a sentinel lymph node test. This test is done to see if the cancer has spread to any lymph nodes. During this test, a dye is injected. Somehow, depending on how this dye reacts, the surgeon can tell if the cancer has spread to the lymph nodes or not. Let me just say, I have really been spared a lot of pain in my lifetime. I have given birth to two children, but other than that, I can't recall many other excruciating experiences I have suffered…until this test. Dr. Fischer had given me a pill to take the morning of the surgery in order to relax me in preparation for this test, but if I had known the extent of the pain I would have to endure during this procedure, I would have asked for something a little stronger…or a whole bottle of something a little stronger. I am convinced that a better way to check for lymph node involvement in breast cancer patients has not been discovered because few men actually develop breast cancer, so they blessedly avoid having to experience the torture of this test. I dare say, those unfortunate enough to develop testicular cancer do not have to go through anything close to as painful as the sentinel node test. The only good thing I can say about this procedure is that it showed that I did not have any lymph node involvement. Praise God. I view this as a miracle because based on the size of my tumor, the fact that there was no lymph node involvement was almost unheard of. God does answer prayers!

Then it was time for the surgery. I hugged my parents, children, and Tim. We all told each other that we loved one another, and then I was rolled away for surgery. I remember being back in the holding room, waiting for the surgery to begin. Dr. Fischer came by to check on me before my anesthesia was started. He made a small talk and told me everything was going to be okay, and then he held my hand and had prayer with me. I knew then I was going to come through the surgery just fine.

Many friends and family gathered in the waiting room while I had surgery. Church friends, childhood friends, family friends, and loved ones took their time that day to be there for my family and me. I will be eternally grateful. Cousins kept my Rachel entertained during the day, so she wouldn't worry so much. My very best life-long friend, Britt Mitchell, helped Claudia write a speech for school that helped keep her occupied. My friend, Dawn Aldridge, acted as the hostess of the waiting room with her basket full of treats. She even thought to bring a book to record the names of friends and family who brought gifts and goodies for my family and me so that I could write thank you notes later. Yes, she is that kind of person. I want to be like her when I grow up. I wish I could have been in the waiting room because it sounded like everyone had a great time. I never dreamed I could draw such a crowd! Friends were there to talk with Tim and my parents to keep them entertained as well. Our clan took up half of the waiting room that day, and I love each person who took the time to make the effort to support us on that scary day.

After about two hours, Dr. Fischer came out to report to Tim and company that his portion of the surgery was over and had gone well. The tumor, along with a couple of other things, had been removed. Now Dr. Beckenstein would begin his part of the procedure, which was the insertion of the tissue expanders. After another hour or so, Dr. Beckenstein came out to report to Tim and company that his part of the surgery was complete, and it had also gone well. I was being moved to recovery and would be taken to a room soon. At this point, most of the guests at the party in the waiting room dispersed to make their way home. They had heard what they needed to hear, and they had completed their mission of being there to support my family through the day. My family and a couple of close friends made their way to the hospital room to await my arrival.

I remember waking up with a splitting headache. I remember being bound tightly around my chest and tubes coming out of both sides of my body. I remember being in pain. The days after surgery remain a blur. I kept a headache for several days. It was finally concluded that I had a reaction to the anesthesia that was used during surgery, which caused the headache. Then I was getting an anti-nausea medication that exacerbated the headache. It took several days to get all of that sorted out. In the meantime, I felt rotten and let everyone know it! Poor Tim was the person who stayed with me during my convalescence at the hospital. Here is when that "for better or worse, for sickness or in health" part of those marriage vows started to really be tested. Thankfully, Tim passed with flying colors. No matter how nasty I got during my drug-induced stupor (yeah, I'll blame it all on the drugs), Tim remained kind and composed. He helped me get up and walk to the restroom, he helped me walk around the halls of the hospital like I was instructed, and he talked to the nurses in a nice way when I seemed to come across a little gruff for some reason. I really didn't have time to process what had been done to me during the surgery because I felt so horrible; looking back that may have been a good thing. At least the incredible headache was keeping my mind off of thinking about what the surgery had done to my body. The day finally dawned when I could go home. I was still in terrible shape. In fact, right before I was set to be released, Tim and I were taking one more stroll around the nurse's station, and I threw up right there in the middle of the hallway. Lovely, I know. I really didn't care. I was just ready to get home, even if I had to carry a barf bag with me in the car...and use it.

Our Freezer Runneth Over

Some folks care too much. I think it's called
love.

—A. A. Milne, *Winnie the Pooh*

We slowly, very slowly drove home. I had situated
a small travel pillow between the seatbelt of the
car and myself. I was so thankful that my friend Dawn
had provided this jewel of a gift. Who else would
have thought of such a thing? I felt every bump and
jolt of the car on the journey. I was overjoyed to be
home, but I felt like an infant. I could not lift my arms,
bathe myself, or do much of anything. I had to pretty
much let everyone else completely take care of me. I am
not one of those women who find it impossible to let
others take care of her. In fact, I quite enjoy not doing
anything and letting everyone else do all of the work.
I would have enjoyed it a lot more though, if I had not
been in excruciating pain. The worst things, though,
were the drainage tubes coming out of the sides of my
body. I felt like octo-mom. Not because of the number
of offspring I had but because of the tentacles coming

out of my sides. The purpose of these drains was to siphon liquid out of the sides of my body. The liquid in the drains had to be expelled several times per day, and it had to be measured and recorded. I know it is awful. Guess who this horrible job fell to? Tim, of course. He did it without ever gagging or complaining. I, on the other hand, gagged every time I looked at the drains and had to turn my head when Tim had to do his duty. These drains, like the sentinel lymph node test, I am sure were designed by a man because they just hung down, and they were very heavy. Luckily, my friend Carol, who had been through all of this before, gave me an apron with pockets, specially designed for those tubes to fit in. All I had to do was tie the apron around my waist and tuck the tubes in the pockets. This helped tremendously. Obviously, the apron was designed by a woman.

Once we arrived home, my church family kicked in to high gear. We had been attending White Springs Baptist Church in Rainbow City, Alabama, for about twelve years before my surgery. Our church family had supported us through a miscarriage, the birth of our second daughter, Tim donating a kidney to his niece, and many other prayer requests and praises in between. However, we had never experienced the love and support of a group of godly people like we did during this period of time. One of the most generous ways that we received support was through food. Two friends agreed to head up the food committee. Church members signed up through Angie Mabrey and Dawn Aldridge as to when to provide meals for us. Now, we are a family of four. Tim will eat anything except onions. Rachel is a pretty good eater for an eight-year-old. Claudia eats cereal and chicken. And I will eat absolutely anything, but I felt so rotten during this period of time, I couldn't eat much more than a few crackers. Church members dutifully signed up to bring meals. They would usually call the day before to make arrangements. The conversation would generally go something like this: "Tonya, what would you like to eat tomorrow?" church lady would ask.

"We really have plenty. If you just want to bring some chicken, that would be great," Tonya would say.

"Chicken? Are you sure? That is all you want? What about some dessert?"

"No, really. We have five cakes from the last five meals. Chicken would be great. Tim, Claudia, and Rachel all love chicken."

"Well, I hate to just bring chicken. What about macaroni and cheese or mashed potatoes?"

"I promise, we have so much. Chicken will be fine. We would love chicken."

"If you are sure, I'll bring it by about noon tomorrow, if that's okay."

"That will be great. Thanks so much."

The next day at noon, church lady arrives with fried chicken, baked chicken, chicken fingers, chicken livers, chicken casserole, chicken and rice, macaroni and cheese, mashed potatoes and gravy, green beans, corn, tomatoes, rolls, cornbread, coleslaw, apple pie, a chocolate cake, and a gift card to KFC. "I thought you were just bringing chicken. This is too much," Tonya would say as she attempted to make eye contact over the pile of dishes balancing in church lady's arms.

"Don't be silly," church lady would chuckle. "We love ya'll so much, and this is the least I could do."

That is how it is done in the South, I guess. When we can't do anything else, we can cook; and in a situation like mine, love and food just naturally went together. I honestly do not understand how people are able to get through difficult situations in life without the love and support of a church family. The prayers, phone calls, cards, supportive words, acts of kindness, and of course the food, meant more than can ever be expressed. I hate to admit it, but until I had breast cancer, my family had never eaten so well!

Lazy Days of Recovery

Sometimes you're the windshield; sometimes you're the bug.

—Mark Knopfler, "The Bug"

As I began to recover, I had to make weekly trips to Birmingham to see Dr. Fischer and Dr. Beckenstein. After the discharge from the octo-tubes reached a certain level, Dr. Beckenstein took the awful tubes out. A week or so later, the stitches came out. I slowly began to feel a little better. I won't lie, I couldn't keep up with my family's washing or manage to keep my house clean, but I couldn't do those things before the surgery either, so that was nothing new. As I began feeling better, I started being able to spend more days by myself. I have always enjoyed my alone time, and as a mom, that can be hard to come by sometimes. Those first few days by myself were quite enjoyable. I still could not do any strenuous jobs, so sitting around on the couch all day watching TV was fine. I didn't feel guilty about doing it. However, after awhile, I could only take so much of Kathie Lee and Hoda. There are only so many hours of daytime programming that a body can stand. Here is a list of the ways I began spending my days:

Top 10 Ways I Spent My Days Recovering:

10. Woke up and read *The Gadsden Times* from cover to cover.

9. Reread *The Gadsden Times* just in case I missed something.

8. Watched *Chopped*.

7. Watched *Chopped-All-Stars*.

6. Started thinking about lunch and wondering what four unrelated ingredients I could put together to make something yummy.

5. Ate lunch.

4. Watched for the mailman to arrive.

3. Rushed out to check mail and read cards that friends had sent. I put aside all of those pesky hospital bills for Tim to deal with another day.

2. Waited for Rachel, Claudia, and Tim to get home and asked way too many questions about how their days went.

1. Counted my many blessings!

Yes, this schedule was stimulating and fun for about a week, but then it did begin to get old. But I didn't have to wait long for another form of fun to begin—my weekly "pump it up parties" at Dr. Beckenstein's office. During surgery, Dr. Beckenstein had inserted tissue expanders. The time had now come to begin expanding the expanders. Once a week, Tim and I went to Dr. Beckenstein's office to have saline injected into the expanders. This procedure sounds simple enough, but I felt like one of those giant balloons in the Macy's Thanksgiving Day Parade every time I left the office. The difference was not visible, but I felt like I was "floating" after each visit. Again, I was thankful that I had the opportunity to be treated by Dr. Beckenstein and begin to start getting my feminine "shape" back, but this was a painful and uncomfortable process. I would ask Tim after each of these visits if I looked like the Pillsbury doughboy, but he assured me that that was all in my imagination. I wasn't so sure that I believed him though. I just knew that I was going to start to float away after one of these visits, and Tim was going to have to run after me to try to catch my pant leg and try to pull me back down to planet earth.

Thanks, Raquel

Sometimes good things fall apart so better things can fall together.

—Marilyn Monroe

On one particular day, Tim and I had set off to Birmingham with two stops in mind. I had an appointment at my favorite plastic surgeon's office, but first, I wanted to stop by a place that a fellow "sister of the pink ribbon society" had told me about. That particular store catered to cancer patients, and they did wig fittings. Everyone who had been through this before me had stressed the importance of shopping for a wig before your hair began to fall out in order to match color, texture, and style. For some strange reason, I thought wig shopping sounded fun, like playing dress-up, like something I would really enjoy! However, as soon as I sat down in the chair, and the lady put the first wig on me, I burst into tears. It didn't help that the wig was gray and styled in the fashion of Betty White. Not flattering at all to say the least! The nice lady quickly jerked that one off my head and looked around some more. After we both calmed down a bit, she finally presented several wigs that were more age or style appropriate (ha, ha as if), and I settled on one. Unfortunately, it was platinum blonde. I thought I could pull it off, but I wasn't sure how the little ladies from church would react if I walked in on Sunday as a platinum blonde. Actually, they would probably respond with, "You go, girl!"

Finally, we turned to the catalog. Now in the catalog, you get to look at Raquel Welch in her body hugging black sweaters as she models all of the wigs. This is something that the "sisters of the pink ribbon society" just *love* to see. I looked at wigs with names like "flirt," "vibrant," and "center stage." They looked fabulous on Raquel, but even the best one I tried on that day ended up just looking like a rabbit fur coat on my head. I decided right then that if I did get a wig, I was going to name mine "Thumper."

After about an hour and a half of trying on wigs and wiping tears away, I decided on a style that I thought looked similar to my current hairstyle, which I lovingly referred to as my hair helmet. The nice lady from the store ordered it for me in two different colors. Once they came in, I could decide which one I liked best. I waited patiently for a few days and then received the call that the wigs were in. Of course, I had some kind of appointment in Birmingham the next day anyway, so Tim and I set off to pick up my new hair.

I remained hopeful that once I had a wig that was the right style and color, it would look better than the other options I had tried on. It is hard to imagine how a style will look in the correct hue when you are too busy concentrating on the fact that you are suddenly transformed into a redhead for a moment. And blondes do not have more fun if they are wearing a wig and sitting in a chair at a cancer store waiting for their hair to fall out, just saying.

Finally, the lady unveiled my two options. Two brand-new Raquel wigs, one slightly darker than the other, both styled as close to a hair helmet as I have ever seen. Let me just say, I was less than overjoyed. I carefully tried on each option. We combed, shook, worked, sprayed, and fussed. Finally, I had each wig whipped into shape, at least a shape that looked like my normal hair. I tried one on and then the other and then switched back again. I finally settled on the lighter of the two. I put it on one more time and looked in the mirror. Yep, there I sat with a big ole rabbit fur coat right on top of my head. I had reservations about just how happy "Thumper" and I were going to be together. I was afraid I would probably have a better chance of looking like Raquel in a tight black sweater than looking good in my new hair. Fat chance.

One Can Never Be Too Early

You were given this life because you were strong
enough to live it.

—Author Unknown

Dr. Fischer had prepared me that I would most
likely need chemotherapy and radiation after my
surgery. The chemotherapy was necessary for the type
of cancer I had, and the radiation was due to the size
of my tumor. My tumor was so large that it was right
at the cut-off point of going ahead with radiation as
an added precaution against recurrence of cancer. Dr.
Fischer said he would leave that decision up to my
oncologist. So now, we got to add a new doctor to the
mix. My friend, stalker, nurse, guardian angel, had done
her research and come up with the name of Dr. James
Cantrell. According to all of Ashley's sources, Dr.
Cantrell was *the* oncologist to see. Dr. Fischer made the
referral, and I soon had my first appointment with Dr.
Cantrell at the Bruno Cancer Center at St. Vincent's.
I was very nervous about my first visit to the Bruno
Cancer Center. I was afraid I would see pitiful people
in pitiful pain in pitiful situations. Mostly though, I saw

people from all walks of life who had been blindsided by stupid cancer like I had. They were just like Tim and me, doing everything they could to get through this horrible experience and get on with their lives. Tim and I liked Dr. Cantrell immediately. He was a no nonsense kind of doctor who gave us the facts and didn't waste our time. The first step in this chemotherapy journey would be to have a port inserted for the medicine to be injected through. So I made an appointment for the port to be put in place by Dr. Fischer, my super-surgeon.

Leave it to a hospital to make a procedure that takes twenty minutes to consume half of the day. My parents eagerly agreed to accompany me for this procedure. I pride myself on being a person who arrives promptly to appointments. On good days, mostly those good days were before the arrival of my children, I can make it ten to fifteen minutes early to a designated engagement. This trait was definitely taught to me by my parents. I was supposed to be at the hospital by 5:00 a.m. for the port insertion procedure, and we arrived promptly at the hospital at 3:15 a.m. Just in case traffic was bad or something unimaginable happened like Jesus coming back, that would make us run late. I guess in case of the Second Coming, Daddy would have told Jesus we had to make a detour by St. Vincent's on the way to heaven. Some people live by the motto, "You can never be too rich or too thin." My parents live by the motto, "You can never arrive too early to an event or eat dinner too early in the day." Anyway, we got to St. Vincent's with hours to spare. No apocalypse that particular morning. The procedure went fine, and we found ourselves pulling out of the hospital parking lot at eleven. At least it was 11:00 am and not 11:00 pm. Just in time for a delicious dinner at Cracker Barrel at a reasonable hour. Apparently, my parents had eaten lunch at around 6:30 a.m. in the hospital dining room while I was having my procedure done.

Hospital time exists in another dimension. No one got in a hurry once their feet touched hospital ground. I truly think my Rachel has a career in the medical field in her future because even now nothing can light a fire under her. I have had to pray for forgiveness long before the altar call on many Sunday mornings because of my less than Christlike reaction to finding Rachel still in her pajamas in her bedroom when the rest of the family is ready to run out the door for Sunday school. She never gets in a hurry or worries about being late while her older sister, Claudia, and I rush, rush, rush to get places half an hour early. Maybe it's a birth-order thing, but then again, I don't think an entire hospital is run by the last in birth order (nice way of saying babies).

After the procedure, recovery, and chest x-ray, I still had time to watch a couple of episodes of *Say Yes to the Dress* while waiting to be dismissed. So the day wasn't a total downer. I do believe God was also trying to teach me patience through this journey. I was discovering there was a lot of "hurry up and wait" that had to be tolerated to get to the final result. Dr. Fischer was great as always. He had even come back to the hospital room to talk to me before I was dismissed. This was after he had already spoken to my parents following the procedure. God definitely led me to the right surgeon. Things were moving along at a remarkable pace. Next step…chemotherapy.

Diet Coke, Snickers, and Taxotere

Experience is not what happens to you. It's
what you do with what happens to you.

—Rick Warren,
The Purpose Driven Life:
What on Earth Am I Here For?

Chemotherapy. Is there a more dreaded word in the
English language to hear? Well, I guess *death*; and
that might have been what I had been facing had I not
gone forward with chemotherapy, so I decided to just
make the best of it. My chemotherapy would be on
Wednesdays, spaced three weeks apart. I was uneasy as
Tim and I made our way to the Bruno Cancer Center
for that first treatment. We had no idea of what to
expect at that first visit. Would I become violently ill and
throw-up all the way home? Would my hair start falling
out in chunks as I was walking out the door? Would I
ever be the same after this poison entered my body?
This was probably the most apprehensive that I had

been since this whole process had started. I mean, why yell "Boo" at Halloween when yelling "Chemotherapy" works just as well? I guess because "Boo" is shorter, but really, both scare the heck out of you!

We parked our car and made our way inside the building. Much effort had gone into trying to make the waiting room of the Bruno Cancer Center as comfortable as possible. There was a big fish tank with lots of little Nemos and Dorys swimming around in an effort to lull visitors into a calm state of mind by watching their graceful gliding through the water. There was always a jigsaw puzzle available for working. Recliners were available for relaxation. Television sets were mounted and tuned to various stations for the viewing pleasure of patients and caregivers alike. However, nothing could change the fact that we were all there for the same reason—chemotherapy.

Tim and I patiently waited, and then the nurse finally called my name. At first, I just went back by myself to a little holding room. Here my weight and vital signs were checked. Then the nurse was ready to insert the needle into my port. My port had just been put in place a few days earlier, so the site was still pretty tender. The nurse sprayed some kind of freezing spray on the site and then prepared to insert the needle. She told me to take a deep breath, she counted to three, and then she stuck. It wasn't too bad. I guess I was numb from the freezing spray, but so far this wasn't as dreadful as I had imagined. A short tube was connected to the needle. This is where the medications would be attached. I was sent back to the waiting room with

Tim for a few minutes until I was called back to the treatment area.

Tim was looking at the needle stuck in my port, asking me if it was too painful, when my name was called again to go back to the treatment area. This was it. I was about to receive chemotherapy for the first time. If I had imagined a thousand things that may have happened to me in my lifetime, chemotherapy would not have been on the list, but here we were. We walked slowly down the hall to the treatment room. The treatment room was an L-shaped room with little areas separated by partitions. In each little area, there was a giant reclining chair with an attached tray. Over the chair was a TV that could be tuned into whatever show the patient wanted to watch. Why should a girl have to miss the daily deal on QVC or get behind on her stories just because she was enduring chemotherapy? There was an outlet in each cubby, so computers and cell phones or other devices could be plugged in and charged during treatment. There was a bookshelf in the treatment room that was packed with books that may be of interest to patients or those caregivers who had accompanied patients to treatment. There was also an area with drinks, ice, and snacks available to have during treatment. Huh, I suddenly started thinking this may not be so bad after all. Let's see, I will be confined to one place for at least three hours or more. I will not be able to, or expected to, do anything else like fold laundry, cook, load the dishwasher, or help with homework. I can have any snack I want hand delivered to me by my loving husband. I can read a good book, watch TV, or nap without being interrupted. This chemotherapy thing was beginning to sound better and better. If I had to do it, I might as well enjoy it, right?

The nurse talked to us and gave us lots of information and papers. I honestly didn't hear much. I was already planning my first snack and activity. I thought I would go with a Snickers and a good Frank Peretti book to start off. I needed a little adventure. I sat down in the chair, and she brought out the medicine bags. I would be given a lovely cocktail of Taxotere and Cytoxan. Those were the two anti-cancer chemotherapy drugs that would help ensure that I would have no recurrence of cancer. I would also be administered an anti-nausea medication. The first bag was hung on the IV stand and hooked up to my port, and my chemo therapy session began. I thought I would feel burning or pain of some sort, but I actually didn't feel anything. I didn't even know anything at all was happening, much less the war that was being fought inside my body between the good drugs and the bad cells. I relaxed a little. Tim stayed back in the treatment room with me long enough for me to get situated and to feel comfortable, and then he moved back to the waiting room to stay until the three- to four-hour treatment was over. Before he left, I asked for a Diet Coke and the Peretti book. I settled in for the duration.

Periodically, Tim came back to the treatment room to check on me. Dr. Cantrell stopped by to talk with us. I had my Diet Coke, book, asked for a Snickers, asked for some cheese crackers, napped, sent some text messages, and finally, about four hours later, my first chemotherapy session was over. The nurse removed the needle from my port, gave us some parting instructions, and we were on our way. If this was all that chemotherapy consisted of, I wanted to sign up for once a week at least! I could relax with no interruptions, read a whole book without losing it six times before I finally finished it, and have an entire TV to myself without having to watch Disney channel or ESPN for hours at a time! This was wonderful! Why did people say chemotherapy was bad?

Chemotherapy Is Bad!

Life's problems wouldn't be called 'hurdles' if there wasn't a way to get over them.

—Author Unknown

Since college, I had experienced bad headaches, but it was not until my oldest daughter, Claudia, and I had gone to a "Mom and Me" church camp together several years earlier that I experienced my first full-blown migraine. I remember being in a cabin with about ten other moms and daughters, trying to sleep when I first started getting a headache. I had failed to bring any over the counter medication with me on the weekend trip. As we got up the next day and began to go about our activities, my headache got worse and worse. Thankfully, we were leaving that day, so I didn't have to wait too long before we headed home, but it was a long ride home on the church van with five girls, three other mothers, and me with a splitting headache. I discovered that if I grabbed a handful of my hair right on the top of my head and pulled it straight up, it helped ease the pain a little for some reason, so that is how I rode for the trip home, pulling my hair straight up off of my head. When Claudia and I finally made it to our car, I carefully steered with one hand while still pulling my hair with the other until we made it safely home. I am glad no policemen saw us and pulled us over on that little trip, or I may have gotten a ticket for domestic abuse to myself. When I could finally stagger into the house, I immediately took some pain reliever, which immediately came right back up, and then I went to bed. I spent the rest of that day and night throwing up and pulling my hair, trying to get some relief from the headache. When it finally subsided a little, I called my doctor. He then referred me to a neurologist, who did all of the tests necessary to confirm the diagnosis of migraine headaches. I have been on preventative medication ever since that time. Thankfully, I have never experienced a headache as bad as the one I got on the camping trip, until the one I got after my first chemotherapy treatment.

It started on the sixty-mile drive home. I felt fine when Tim and I left the hospital, very relaxed even. But the longer we drove, the worse I felt. I could tell what was coming. I knew it was going to be a full-blown migraine. And boy, oh boy, was I right. By the time we made it home, I was pulling my hair and racing for the bathroom. I thought I might not have to wait for chemotherapy to make my hair fall out because if the headache didn't go away, I was going to pull all of it out after treatment number one. I tried taking my preventative medication and then another medication that my neurologist had given me in case I ever got a

migraine. Both of those medicines came right back up.
I tried taking some of the pain medication I had from
my surgery. Finally, that knocked me out. I was able to
sleep for awhile, but when that medicine would wear
off and I would wake up, the headache would be just as
bad. Tim called the Cancer Center the next morning to
ask for some help. The nurse he talked to assured him
that this was not an unusual side effect. Didn't we read
about it in the literature that was provided? No, I was
too busy eating my candy bar and reading my Christian
fiction to be bothered with informational literature. I
had to use my four hours of "me" time wisely. I didn't
want to waste it thinking about things like cancer! Now
I know I was taking chemotherapy at the time, but I do
have a vivid imagination, and I was working with what
I had.

The nurse assured Tim she would make a note
in my chart that the headache was probably caused
by the anti-nausea medication administered during
chemotherapy. She said during the next treatment, they
would use a different medication that would probably
not cause a headache as a side effect. Great. That
would help next time, but I was still suffering this time.
I continued to rest and complain, take medicine and
complain until the headache finally began to subside.
But it did last several days, and it made me nervous
about the other chemotherapy sessions to come. Even
four hours of uninterrupted "me" time was not worth
having to deal with a skull-crushing migraine every
three weeks.

After each chemotherapy treatment, I also had to get a Neulasta shot the following day. Neulasta is a drug that boosts the body's ability to produce white blood cells to fight off infection during chemotherapy. I had worked it out with my insurance company and Dr. Cantrell's office to have the shot sent to my house. That way, I wouldn't have to drive all the way back to Birmingham the day after chemotherapy just to get a shot. My good friend, Rita King, who is a nurse and works in the school system with me, agreed to administer the Neulasta shot after each chemotherapy treatment. I was so thankful that Rita had agreed to take on this responsibility. It gave me more time to recover from each treatment without having to make the one-hundred and twenty or so mile round-trip back to the Cancer Center for one shot. Rita is a walking ray of sunshine, and she always made me feel better by her mere presence; however, the shot had some nasty side effects of its own to leave behind.

I won't go into extreme detail here, but let's just say that the Neulasta shot along with the chemotherapy gave me some pretty severe stomach issues. Very severe stomach issues. That would prove to be the case after each chemotherapy treatment. No matter what I did to prepare for the treatment, things would just come to a standstill after that Neulasta shot. No amount of Fiber-One, apples, and Raisin Bran would do the trick, even when they were eaten all together between two pieces of whole grain toast with prunes between each layer and washed down with a tall glass of Metamucil. It was just terrible. I certainly know it could have been worse. I have heard the horror stories of people who were not able to eat at all the whole time they were taking chemotherapy, and of some people who were nauseated the entire time they were having treatment. I know I had it pretty easy with just a migraine and some tummy trouble, but it still royally stunk.

To Wig or Not to Wig,
That Is the Question

Sometimes the things we can't change end up
changing us for the better.

—Jieho Lee, *The Air I Breathe*

I had been expecting this heart-wrenching hour
since the day the doctor told me that I had cancer.
I think every woman who gets the diagnosis begins to
dread it the moment she hears that she will have to
endure chemotherapy. I was waiting for it to happen.
My friend Carol told me that losing her hair was
probably the hardest thing she had to deal with when
she went through chemotherapy, so I had been trying
to mentally prepare myself for some time. I thought I
was ready. Now that fateful day had finally arrived—
the day I lost my hair. It began gradually on Saturday
when I noticed a few more strands than usual in the
bathtub drain after my shower. Then on Sunday, there
were even more there. By Monday, I could literally run
my hand through my hair and end up with a fistful of

brown tendrils tangled around my fingers. Rachel just loved this trick. On Tuesday, I looked like Pigpen from *Peanuts*, only it was a trail of hair in my wake, not trash. I actually could not walk without my hair falling out. So I made an appointment with my hairdresser to go have it all shaved off. I thought if I took a proactive approach, I could remain in control and thus handle the situation with a bit more composure. I felt even better when I talked to my stylist, Krystal, on the phone, and she told me she now had half of her head shaved, so we could be "twinsies." Oh, to be young and be doing this for a fashion statement!

Tim offered to go with me to the salon and provide support, but as sweet as the offer was, I told him I wanted to do this by myself. Beauty salons are something women do by themselves. I've cried in the chair before, so it wouldn't be a new experience for me. I've had bad perms, too short cuts, off kilter dye jobs, and the list could go on and on and on...This would not be the first time for me to shed tears over my locks. So I put my "big girl panties" on once again and headed to the beauty shop. I sat down in the chair, took a deep breath, and told Krystal to start. Krystal was so sweet as she sheared and made small talk about "normal things" just like she always did. She didn't talk about cancer, surgeries, or hospitals. She asked about my girls and my job and told me about her little boy. To the casual observer, we probably looked like the typical stylist and client (except I was a little old to be getting a punk cut like Krystal's just for the heck of it). Before I knew it, I began to look like G.I. Tonya. But the best part was I didn't shed a single tear. Honestly, not one tear.

The more Krystal shaved, the better I felt about things. It didn't bother me nearly as much as I thought it would (it helped that I wasn't nearly as gray under there as I expected to be either). I even walked out of the salon bareheaded. I had taken a scarf to wear out, but I didn't even bother putting it on. And that sweet Krystal, she didn't even charge me for her services. What a blessing she was to me that day. Hair…is it really that big of a deal? Not considering everything else my family had been through. So I guess I was ready for the whole hair loss thing after all. But now came the hard part. I never dreamed this next issue would cause so much heartache within the Reid household.

Rachel knew that I had made an appointment to have my head shaved on that particular day, so she had begged and pleaded to ride the school bus home that afternoon. I think she was scared to death that I would show up to pick her up at school with my bald head shining in all its glory. I had told her I would do my very best not to embarrass her once I lost my hair. I told her that I would do whatever she wanted me to do to make this easier for her. If that meant wearing a wig, I would wear a wig. If that meant wearing a scarf, I would wear a scarf. If that meant going bald, I would go bald. To which she quickly placed her hand on her hip and stated matter-of-factly, "Uh, bald is *not* an option." I guess she made that perfectly clear.

Let me just say that Rachel did not react favorably to my shaved head. I may not have shed tears over my shorn locks, but my poor eight-year old Rachel did. After showing her my bare head, she wanted me to immediately put my wig on. She made me promise not to leave the house without "Thumper" firmly in place on top of my head. I think she would have preferred that I sleep in the wig so that there was absolutely no chance whatsoever of anyone seeing me au natural. I think her initial reaction (which was crying, crying, and oh yes, more crying) was not so much to the loss of hair as to everything that has been going on. The loss of hair was really the first visual sign that I was really sick. Also, lots of feelings had probably been building up for awhile, and then her seeing me without hair was just the straw that broke the camel's back, hence her reaction to my shaved head.

I tried to love "Thumper." I really, really did. But it just wasn't meant to be. Our relationship started out fine, but then he just didn't hold up his side of the bargain. I refer to Thumper as "he" because he behaved just like a man. When I would put him on my head and proceed to fuss, muss, cry, wail, look in the mirror, and demand to know why I felt so ugly. Sorry, ladies, but you know on those bad, bad days it always gets to ugly. He would just sit there motionless and stare back at me with no response whatsoever to make the situation any better. Now doesn't that sound just like a man to you?

Anyway, I wore Thumper for a total of two whole days. I just couldn't stand to look at myself with him on my head. I knew people knew I was bald underneath there, and no matter what I did, I thought it looked like a wig just crouching there on top of my head. I also had a great aunt who used to wear wigs, and I thought I favored Aunt Sugar a little too much every time I looked in the mirror. Now based on old photographs, Aunt Sugar was once quite a looker; however, when I knew her and saw her with her wigs on, she was usually bossing my mother around or favoring my little sister over me, so those were not good memories to stir up at this emotional time. The wig was pretty, the right color, and the right cut, but I just didn't feel like myself when I had it on. I know it was just me being weird about it, but it was not the right thing for me. I decided to try some "Thumper" alternatives. I started wearing scarves, head-wraps, and hats. For some reason, I felt much more comfortable in those. I know they garnered more attention, but for some reason, they worked for me.

Soon I was buying and borrowing every sort of scarf and head-wrap I could find. I would wrap anything I could find around my head. I started to feel like Carol Burnett that time she portrayed Scarlett O'Hara and had the curtain rod running across her shoulders when she made her dress out of the drapes. I was not above trying a table cloth, blanket, or robe on for a turban. If I thought a design or material would match an outfit, it was fair game. I did have some favorites though. Rita who came and gave me my Neulasta shot after each chemotherapy treatment had a daughter whose family had recently moved to France as missionaries. Her sweet daughter sent me a beautiful hat all the way from France! I adored it and felt so chic when I wore it. Also, a principal at one of the schools where I worked, Mrs. Donna Johnson, had taken a tour of the holy land years earlier and bought a beautiful black and silver pashmina. She gave it to me as gift. I especially liked to wear it to church and on special occasions when I needed to dress up. It was really lovely.

It took a little convincing, but Rachel was eventually okay with my decision to shun "Thumper" in favor of scarves. When she asked me if she could have the wig to play with since I was not going to be wearing it, I felt like we had made great strides. 1 Peter 3:3-4 says "Your beauty should not come from outward adornment, such as braided hair and the wearing of gold jewelry and fine clothes. Instead, it should be that of your inner self, the unfading beauty of a gentle and quiet spirit, which is of great worth in God's sight." We all know that outward appearances are not what matters. Now, I enjoyed a good hair day as much as any woman, but I realized that through the process of losing my hair and living without it for awhile, God was going to really be reminding me of this fact, and I hoped a certain little third grader would also come to understand that too!

Claudia was really amazing about the whole hair loss situation. Her maturity was just incredible. I can say with certainty that I was not even close to her level of maturity when I was her age. In fact, when I was a seventh grader, my mother was my English teacher. One day she dared to speak to me in class…the nerve. That was the maddest I have ever been at her…because she spoke to me in *her* class. Now there's some maturity for ya! I was embarrassed for her to speak to me at school, yet Claudia never even blinked when I would come walking up to her and a group of her friends with my latest chemo bonnet on. *Wow!* I am so thankful God did not see fit to repay me in kind for my own past behavior!

In an effort to remain positive, I decided to make a Top 10 List of Reasons Why Being Hairless Isn't So Bad:

10. You don't have to worry about catching lice.

9. Split ends are a thing of the past.

8. No more worries about seriously mangled at home eyebrow waxing jobs (Come on, ladies, I can't be the only one who has done this).

7. You won't be wasting hours at the drugstore trying to decide between Medium Ash Brown and Medium Golden Brown for that big change you need in your life.

6. No more listening to Rachel complain about finding my stray hair in her precious "Tangle Teaser."

5. No more bad hair days…only no hair days.

4. No more helmet hair (my nickname for my previous hairstyle, and believe me, I use the term "style" loosely).

3. I can finally be cool like Sinead O'Conner. You have to keep in mind that I was a teenager in the 80s when she was the coolest thing around for about five minutes with her bald head.

2. No hairspray…no problem.

1. No more shaving my legs! (Summertime, where art thou?)

The Third Time's a Charm

We are healed from suffering only by experiencing it to the full.

—Marcel Proust

"Wig," Tim said as he slyly motioned toward a little lady walking by us in the waiting room.

"Yep, wig," I agreed.

"Hair."

"Are you sure?" I whispered to my husband Tim as we tried to glance discreetly at the stylishly dressed woman sweeping past us on her way to the treatment room. "I think I remember her from the last time we were here, and if I recall, she was a blonde three weeks ago. Now she is a brunette. I think that proves she is definitely wearing a wig."

"Maybe you're right," conceded Tim, "but it sure looks like real hair to me. That is one of the best wigs I've seen yet. Maybe you should ask her where she shopped for her hair."

"I'll pass. Thank you very much." End of conversation. Tim knew what a sore spot the whole wig or scarf had been for me. I had settled on scarves, and I was sticking with that decision. No looking back for this girl.

Tim and I were sitting in the Bruno Cancer Center at St. Vincent's Hospital in Birmingham awaiting my third chemotherapy treatment, playing hair or wig. This was one of the games we had invented as a way to pass the endless number of hours we found ourselves since my diagnosis of breast cancer. We now had to wait in doctor's offices, wait during chemotherapy, wait for test results, wait in traffic, wait, wait, and wait. We had to do something to entertain ourselves, so we didn't kill each other while we were spending so much quality time together these days.

Today was to be one of the good days though. It was to be my third and last chemotherapy treatment. We arrived at the Cancer Center and waited… waited….and waited. Finally, an hour and a half after my scheduled appointment time, I heard my name called, and I made my way back to the treatment area. Tim always accompanied me and helped me get settled in before he made his way back to the waiting room, for, you guessed it, more waiting. I located my lounge chair and got settled in for the next three hours or so. I always packed a bag to bring along filled with my favorite snacks, books, and magazines to help me pass the time. The nurse hooked up the first bag of medicine to the port that had been surgically implanted into the upper right side of my chest, and I started my chemotherapy. Shortly thereafter, my oncologist came by to see me. We chatted as I sent Tim a text telling him to come back to the treatment room to talk to the doctor too. I told Dr. Cantrell that I was excited that this was my last treatment. To which he replied, "No, this is not your last treatment."

I said, "You said three."

He said, "I said six."

Tim walked up at this time, saw my face, and figured out what was going on. Tim said, "You said three."

"I said six." Dr. Cantrell flipped through my chart and showed us where his report said six treatments spaced three weeks apart. Now, for those who know me well, know I do not have a great memory (okay, not even a good memory); that was why I had made *sure* that somebody had been with me at every appointment. I had been so afraid that I would miss something or hear something wrong. However, Tim and I *both* had heard three treatments spaced three weeks apart. Tim even wrote it down (thanks to Dawn, my highly organized friend who sent me little notepads specifically for this reason)! Dr. Cantrell said maybe he had misspoken. Who knows? All I know is that I thought my chemo days would be over after this treatment, and I had just found out that I would have to go through three more. This was beyond frustrating and very embarrassing! Let's just say I had barely managed to stop myself from hiring a brass band to welcome me home from my thought-to-be-last chemo treatment. That is the kind of celebration I wanted when Tim and I rolled into our driveway after this appointment, and now I had to tell everyone, "Oops, three more to go." I know, that was just the devil and pride working against me, but it still ticked me off, big time!

To sum up how I felt, I thought I would quote a great literary heroine of our time, Ramona, from that much revered work, *Ramona & Beezus* (well, from the movie version anyway), "I'm gonna say a bad word…a really, really, really, bad word…here it comes…Guts! Guts! *Guts!*" I know that three more treatments was not the end of the world. Thankfully, the first treatments had not been too terribly bad, so I had no reason to think that the last ones would be any different. I knew God had a plan, and that everything happened for a reason. I remembered when all of this started, and I thought that I just had three treatments, making the remark that I could do anything three times. Maybe God knew I could only handle chemotherapy treatments in three installments at a time. I was reminded of the verse when Joseph says to his brothers, "You intended to harm me, but God intended it for good to accomplish what is now being done, the saving of many lives" (Genesis 50:20). Well, I say to the devil, "You intended to harm me, but God intended it for good to accomplish what is now being done, the saving of *my* life." Take that evil one! I know something good is going to come out of this. And if the devil doesn't like it he can…I'm gonna say a bad word…a really, really, really bad word…

Happy New Year…a Little Late

Having a place to go–is a home. Having someone to love–is a family. Having both–is a blessing.

—Donna Hedges

It took me a few days to get over the events of that terrible, horrible, no good, very bad day that surrounded my third chemotherapy treatment. I finally came to terms with the fact that I would, in fact, face three more chemotherapy treatments. I could handle that. God had gotten me through all of this cancer craziness so far; he certainly won't leave me hanging now. The Bible tells us in 1 Thessalonians 5: 16–18, "Rejoice always, pray continually, give thanks in all circumstances; for this is God's will for you in Christ Jesus." I must say I was still struggling with the giving thanks for the cancer thing and all, but I did realize I had so, so, so, so much to be thankful for. I once again decided to focus on the positive, and put my "big girl panties" on once again and move forward.

After that first awful chemotherapy treatment that was followed by the migraine sent straight from the devil himself, the next two treatments had not been too bad. I would take my treatment on a Wednesday. I would feel okay for the rest of that day. Once I took my Neulasta shot on Thursday, I would start to feel pretty lousy. By Friday, I was not much fun to be around, and then I usually spent Saturday in the bed. It wasn't that I was nauseous or in excruciating pain. I just felt yucky, so it was better for my family and me if I just closed the bedroom door and waited for the yuckiness to pass. By Sunday, I was always feeling much better. That was the routine that treatments two and three had followed, and sure enough, treatments four, five, and six followed suit. Not fun but not too horrible either. I still got my three to four hours of alone time while I was taking my treatment, followed by the two and a half days of getting over it. We all learned how to deal with this routine, and then before we could even believe it, my chemotherapy treatments were over.

My last chemotherapy treatment fell just after New Year's, so my family and I decided to postpone our New Year's celebration until after that final chemotherapy treatment was done. My daddy had also just recently completed his radiation treatments, so it just felt like a good time to mark the end of a not so great period in our lives and look forward to better days ahead. On the weekend following that last treatment, we planned a celebration at my house. My mother and daddy, sister, Aundrea, brother-in-law, Chris, and my two nieces, Sara and Lilly, joined Tim, Claudia, Rachel, and me for a New Year's Eve party about two weeks after the actual holiday. The girls and I had fun decorating the house with streamers and balloons, pink of course, and every pink-ribboned bedecked item that I had been gifted with since my diagnosis. And believe me, there were quite a few of those because as soon as you are diagnosed with breast cancer, the pink-ribboned items begin to pour in. We had pink-ribboned key chains, pink-ribboned pencils, pink-ribboned ink pens, pink-ribboned hats, pink-ribboned glasses, pink-ribboned bracelets, pink-ribboned Christmas ornaments, and even a pink-ribboned embellished bird house all arranged down the middle of my dining room table in a lovely center piece display. The only thing missing was the pink-ribboned embellished Halloween pumpkin that my cousin, Amy Hutchison, had made for me in October; but try as I might, I just was not able to keep it from finally rotting right away.

When everyone arrived for the party, we ate pizza and other delicious snacks my mom and sister had brought, which of course included a cake with a big pink ribbon in the center. Yes, we were doing this celebration up right! We toasted the new year to come with sparkling grape juice. Then I had a surprise for everyone. I had ordered Chinese lanterns for us to release (think the boat scene from the movie *Tangled*). Trudie Guffey, a friend from church, had done this with her family and had given me the idea. I had ordered the lanterns and kept them a secret from everyone, even Tim. The night of the party, I played the portion of the movie *Tangled* that shows the sky filled with the

Chinese lanterns. I told my family we were going outside to release lanterns into the sky to represent our family letting go of all of the bad things that the past year had held for us and ushering in a new beginning of good things to come for the fresh, new year. We all put on our coats, scarves, hats (I, of course, already had one on), and gloves, and loaded up. I had gotten permission from Rachel's principal and my friend, Carrie Yancey, to do our release in the big field in front of the elementary school, which was about five miles from our house.

Once we got to the school, we all piled out of our cars and got ready for the release. I had purchased enough lanterns for each person to have one to release on his or her own and then for us to release some together. We laughed and oohed and aahed as the beautiful lanterns floated up in the air and out of our sight, taking with them all of the bad memories of the past year. We said little prayers of thanksgiving and made petitions for a better year to come as we released our colorful lanterns up to the heavens, and they danced out of sight. God even sent us a curious, unexpected passerby to be there to take a family picture of the entire group together on our evening of celebration. We definitely celebrated in style that night!

I Did Not Drive My Motorcycle to Chemo

I base my fashion taste on what doesn't itch.

—Gilda Radner

I work in a school system and am in a school just about every single day of the school year; however, I am not a school teacher. My job is that of a school psychometrist. I am employed through the special education department in my school system, and I administer IQ and achievement tests to children. I also do a lot of paperwork, meetings, and compliance checklists, but testing and working with children is the fun part of the job. When I went back to work shortly after my surgery, it wasn't long until I lost my hair. I had the wig vs. scarf struggle and ultimately decided to go with the scarves. One thing I did have some apprehension about, though, was how the children I worked with would react to my choice. I worried that I may frighten them. After all, most kids from rural Alabama had not seen many gypsy princesses in their lifetimes other than in Disney movies. I wasn't sure how they would react to seeing one in real life. And gypsy princess was what I looked like, in my mind anyway. Mostly, the students had no reaction at all; they just regarded me as they normally had. If they liked school, they liked me. If they didn't like school, they didn't like me. Pretty much typical. The students did the tasks that I asked them to do and never made any comments or showed any kind of reaction toward my head gear for the most part.

One day, though, I was working with a middle school student who had some special needs. She kept looking at my head. I could tell something was brewing. Finally, she asked, "Why have you got that on your head?"

"Well," I replied, "I was sick, and I had to take some very strong medicine to help me get better. The medicine was so strong that it made my hair fall out, so that is why I have this scarf on my head." There. *That wasn't so hard*, I told myself. Surely that explanation was simple enough and thorough enough to satisfy her.

"Really?" She asked, studying my head a bit longer.

"Really," I confirmed.

She sat there for a few minutes, staring at my scarf and then looking back at my face. "Take it off. I want to see!" I quickly put my hands on top of my head for fear that she may just yank my scarf right off, and then she would quickly discover that she really didn't want to see my big bald head after all.

One of my favorite head wraps was a little black number that covered my head and tucked under in the back. It was also bedazzled with little silver sparkles all over it. It was one of my most often worn pieces because it would go with many outfits. I was wearing this particular head adornment one day when I was working with a particularly adorable little kindergarten child. She was very talkative and outgoing, but she never mentioned anything about my head covering.

A few days later, I was talking to her mother. Her mother laughed and told me that after I had worked with her daughter, the little girl was riding in the car and asked her mother if she thought I had ridden my motorcycle to school on the day I saw her. The mother told the little girl, no, that she was pretty sure I had not ridden a motorcycle to school. She asked the little girl why she thought that I may have. The child said that she had just wondered because people who ride motorcycles wear those things on their heads, and I had one on my head the day I worked with her. I thought that was so cute! This little girl was trying to figure out why this woman was wearing something on her head in her school, and the only thing she could relate it to was a person who rides motorcycles. Pretty smart, if you ask me. Who would have ever confused my lovely head covering with a bandana, but an innocent child just trying to make sense of her environment? Precious.

Later that same week however, I was in Cracker Barrel wearing the same little black head covering. I thought I looked very sophisticated in it, with all of its sparkles and basic black and all. I was at the register paying my bill when the cashier looked up and said, "Oh, did you ride your motorcycle today?"

"No, I did not. I don't own a motorcycle," I replied.

"Well, I just thought with your do-rag on and all, that you must have ridden your motorcycle today," she continued with a too bright smile.

"No, and this is not a do-rag. This happens to be a stylish head wrap," I responded through clenched teeth. Having a darling little kindergarten child think my stylish head scarf was what a motorcycle rider might wear is one thing, but clearly, this grown woman should be able to tell the difference.

"Oh, I'm sorry. I just thought that since you had that on your head that maybe you rode your motorcycle. It looks like those bandanas that people who ride motorcycles sometimes wear," she said as her smile faded slightly.

"Well, I don't have a motorcycle. I have cancer. I have lost all of my hair because I am taking chemotherapy. And my scarf does not look like a do-rag. It looks like a very stylish, elegant wig alternative!" I said a little too loudly. I know it was mean, but I had a moment there.

"Oh, I am so sorry," the lady replied as her eyes grew to the size of flying saucers. "Well, it looks good. It really looks nice."

"Yeah, whatever," I said as I took my change. Not my finest moment, I will admit.

"God bless you," the poor cashier said as I walked away.

Looking back, I wish I had handled the situation differently. I now realize that the poor lady was just trying to make conversation and be friendly, but what I had found endearing from a kindergarten child just made me angry from an adult. What can I say? I was in the middle of chemotherapy treatments, and my hormones were going crazy. I could be laughing one moment, and then crying like a baby the next, and then screaming at Tim the next. And when you lose your hair, you have to get accustomed to stares and whispers, but honestly, I think that the cashier asking me that question was like asking a fat lady when her baby was due. You just don't do that. I probably received more attention than I would have if I had gone the wig route, but I just couldn't do that. I guess what made me so angry that day was that in my imagination, I pictured myself looking more like a gypsy princess or an exotic visitor from a far off land. It just hurt my feelings that what I really looked like was a Hells Angel. That was confirmed by two independent judges. I know looking like a motorcycle rider is not a bad thing, but it just wasn't the style I had in mind for myself; however, since I had the headgear already, maybe a big Harley was something I needed to think about for the A.C. (after cancer) years. I had not ridden my motorcycle to chemo, but maybe in the future, I would be riding one to PTA meetings and church. Obviously, I could pull it off. I already had the do-rag to go with one.

Radiate, Rinse, Repeat

There's a crack in everything; that's how the light gets in.

—Leonard Cohen, "Anthem"

After I had finished with my chemotherapy treatments, it was time to think about radiation. I had talked to Dr. Cantrell about the possibility of doing my radiation treatments in Gadsden, since I would be required to have those every day for a long period of time. He said that he had a colleague in Gadsden that he had referred several patients to, and he felt confident in my receiving my radiation treatment closer to home. So I made an appointment to see Dr. Lowndes Harrison at Gadsden Regional Medical Center. The day of the appointment, Tim and I were led into a treatment room, which contained shelf upon shelf of clown dolls. All variety of little clown dolls with porcelain faces were sitting on shelves just staring at Tim and me as we waited for the doctor to come in. We weren't sure if we should laugh or cry.

Finally, Dr. Harrison's nurse came in to go over paperwork. She was so nice that we decided not to let the clowns scare us off. Dr. Harrison was not in at that first appointment, so I had to see a doctor who was covering for him. This doctor basically told me it looked like I would be facing about thirty-five radiation treatments. I went ahead and had my initial scan that day and then went home to wait until I heard from the office as to when I would officially begin these treatments. I got the call a day or two later, and the staff was wonderful about working out a time in the afternoons for me to get my treatments that would be most convenient.

To me, radiation was worse than chemotherapy, simply because I had to go every single day for seven straight weeks, excluding weekends. I would work all day, drive across town to Gadsden Regional, strip naked, put on a hospital gown, have my treatment (which lasted approximately ten minutes), get dressed again, drive back across town, pick up my girls, and then proceed to do whatever afternoon activities they had for whatever day it was. It was completely exhausting. After about the second full week of treatments, the fatigue really started to get to me. I had never been one with loads of energy to begin with, but the radiation was really an energy-zapper.

The actual treatments were not bad at all. I would lie flat on a table and turn my head to the right with my left arm lifted above my head. The Cancer Center had installed tranquil nature scenes on the ceiling and wall to be just in sight when having to hold your head in awkward positions during treatment. Those were nice, but something more along the lines of pictures of Mario Lopez in a Speedo would have done more to get my mind off what was going on than seeing wheat blowing in the breeze. The radiology technician would then line up the giant machine to wherever the magic radiation rays were to hit my body and then leave the room. The machine was then turned on and would send invisible radiation rays to my body as it moved over me. The whole process was painless and quick. I did have to be marked up with black x's on the area where the radiation was administered. I didn't really mind this though. In fact, I kind of felt like a rebel, since this would be the closest I would ever come to getting a tattoo. (I may change my mind if I ever actually go through with getting that Harley.) The radiology guys stuck to x's, even though I would have preferred a butterfly or a pretty flower. Oh well.

My skin did begin to become affected by the radiation toward the end of my treatments. Dr. Harrison and my radiation technician were concerned about one area in particular, so treatments were suspended for a couple of days while my skin healed a bit. The only reason that this really bothered me was that now my treatments would creep into my Spring Break week when the girls and I would both be out of school. I just hated the thought of having to go to treatments during my vacation week too! But, Claudia went on a mission trip with the church to Florida that week, and Rachel spent several days with her grandparents, so what else did I have to do? Might as well go on to radiation. At least it gave me yet another excuse to put off cleaning out my closets.

The Cancer Center at Gadsden Regional was much smaller than that at St. Vincent's, and everyone greeted me by name by the time my treatments were over. The radiation guys and everyone there were very sweet to me, and it was so much more convenient to just drive across town than to have to drive an hour to Birmingham and another hour back home each day for a ten-minute treatment. On the day I finished my treatments, I was presented with a certificate from the Cancer Center commemorating my completion of my treatment cycle. I immediately took a picture of myself holding the certificate giving a thumbs up and posted it on Facebook with the comment, "I went through seven weeks of radiation, and all I got was this crummy certificate…" I was proud of my certificate, my fake tattoos, and my ability to make it through one more phase of this battle with a smile on my face.

A Huge Sigh of Relief

Fall seven times, stand up eight.

—Japanese Proverb

It has now been exactly one year since I first discovered that awful lump. As I think back over all my family and I have gone through in a year's time, it is mind-boggling. After getting over the initial shock of actually having breast cancer and realizing it wasn't a death sentence, merely a bump in the road of my life (maybe a gigantic pothole is a better way to describe it), I had hoped that in one year, everything would be totally back to "normal" for us. While that is not the case, things are slowly but surely returning to the way I remember them. I now have enough hair to go "scarf-less" and not be too self-conscious about it, I now have enough energy to keep up with my girls' after school activity schedules for the most part, and I now can have actual conversations with people who don't always somehow circle back to, you guessed it, cancer. Yes, things are getting better day by day.

I do have some major hurdles still to face, however. I assumed after I completed my radiation treatments, my reconstruction surgery would follow soon after. That has not been the case. Apparently, radiation causes so much harm to the skin, that it takes quite a while for it to become healed enough to endure surgery. So, I am still awaiting my final reconstruction surgery at this point. I dutifully report to my plastic surgeon's office about once per month for him to examine my skin. So far, he has not deemed it "healed." I am so ready to be rid of these tissue expanders and have the final implants in place. The expanders are very uncomfortable and now rather lopsided due to the radiation. Just being honest here. It is impossible to forget all that I have been through when I have the daily reminder of the expanders bringing everything back to the forefront of my memory each morning. It is difficult to explain the sensation of the expanders. Having two giant crockpot lids placed on your chest with an elastic bandage wrapped tightly around you keeping them in place is the closest I can come to describing the feeling. They are very restricting, heavy, and unnatural. I have chosen to refer to the whole expander situation as putting on my "breastplate of righteousness" every day. If I've got to feel this way, I might as well try to make something positive out of it, and I certainly can use extra protection from my armor of God. So, I patiently await what I pray will be my final surgery in this oh so long odyssey.

I also will have to go for blood tests and checkups forever, I guess. I have just recently been for a check-up with Dr. Fischer, and it demonstrated to me how

these visits will probably affect me from now on. Tim
and I went in for a routine check-up. Dr. Fischer was
charming, as usual, and encouraging in all of his pre-exam
conversation. It was finally time for his examination of
me. He examined me, and became a little concerned
when he felt something under my left arm. He probed
and prodded and became more and more concerned.
He assured me that what he was feeling was probably
just fluid buildup from the radiation treatments, but he
said that he would feel better if we did a new PET scan
just to make sure. Not what I was expecting to hear.

A date was scheduled for the test, and Tim and
I headed home. I must admit that I had not gone
exploring my body since my discovery of the tumor a
year ago. I figured that now I saw so many doctors on
such a regular basis that if I had an infected splinter
causing some inflammation, someone would find it
and rule it out as a tumor. But now that Dr. Fischer
had said he felt something under my arm, I couldn't
stop feeling up under there, and of course, now I felt
something too. Even though I had undergone a double
mastectomy, six chemotherapy treatments, seven weeks'
worth of radiation treatments, and negative blood tests
from my oncologist, I was now convinced that I had
a watermelon sized tumor in my left arm pit. All of
those emotions that I had dealt with a year ago came
flooding back. I was once again a total wreck. The
test was scheduled for a Friday, which meant we had
to wait a whole weekend for the results on Monday.
I was already talking to myself about going through
chemotherapy again. I was trying to remind myself

that I had done it one time, and I could do it again. I had to hide from the girls on several occasions that weekend while we awaited the results because we had not told them about the test, and I didn't want them to see me crying like a baby. I would find myself suddenly sobbing while watching Rachel turn cartwheels. I was thinking about all the activities I would miss seeing this year while I fought the cancer battle yet again.

We did not tell my parents or my sister about the test; I kept telling myself that if everything was okay, they did not need to worry unnecessarily. We told the members of our Sunday school class, our pastor, and a few other close friends who we knew would pray. I can't tell you all the scenarios that played through my mind between Friday and Monday. I had hoped that I would hear fairly early in the day on Monday what the verdict was. That way, I could at least start making preparations for Battle Cancer: Round Two. Thankfully, Dr. Fischer called early on Monday morning. He quickly delivered the news that what he felt was merely fluid buildup, and the PET scan showed nothing of concern. Thank you, Lord! I felt like the weight of the world had been lifted off my shoulders. I was beyond happy and relieved. I honestly think I would have taken the news harder the second time around because I now knew what I would have to face, and not just me, but my entire family. I realized many people do not get to feel the relief that I felt. Unfortunately, many times the horrible, awful cancer hangs around and makes repeat appearances at multiple locations where it is most certainly not welcome. I am so thankful that Dr. Fischer does err on the side of caution and checks out any suspicions he may have, and I now know that each time I go in for a routine visit, a little part of me will worry that this may be the time when cancer will rear its ugly head again. I know I can't dwell on that, but I don't know how I could possibly block it out of my mind totally. I guess that is just something we survivors learn to live with. One more thing cancer brings with it when it enters our lives.

James 1:2–4 says, "Consider it pure joy, my brothers and sisters, whenever you face trials of many kinds, because you know that the testing of your faith produces perseverance. Let perseverance finish its work so that you may be mature and complete, not lacking anything." When I was first diagnosed with cancer, joy was the last thing on my mind, but Tim and I both felt it was so important to choose joy as we dealt with this horrible situation. There were many, many days when I felt lots of emotions that were a world away from joy, but I would say that the overarching mood of our family's time during this period was joyful. I am very proud of that fact. What I am not so proud of is my lack of maturity which was quite evident in my reaction to the little scare with my last PET scan. I am just glad that God (and Dr. Beckenstein) aren't finished with me yet!

Part II

Twists and Turns and Some Things I've Learned

Ode to Chemotherapy

'Twas the night before chemo and all through my mind
where worrisome thoughts of this and that kind.

My bag was packed full of things I might need.
I'd even thrown in some books in hopes I may get to read.

The backpacks were hanging on the doorknobs with care,
so we could get the girls off to school with but a minute to spare.

Then Tim in his sweater vest and I in my jeans
headed off to Birmingham to see Dr. Beckenstein's team.

In and out quickly, Tim and I flew,
as Nurse Mandy "pumped me up." She knew just what do!

Next we headed right out the door,
over to the Cancer Center to find out what was in store.

Ports, and needles, and IVs, and such,
At first glance, I thought it might be too much!

Then out of the hallway, there arose such a clatter,
Dr. Cantrell came by to see just what was the matter.

He put me at ease and said, "Don't be upset.
Sit back, relax, and tell the nurses what to get."

So I leaned back in my chair and propped my feet right up,
grabbed my book, some crackers, and asked for Diet Coke
     in a cup.

Once I got the hang of it and learned how to do it,
Chemo wasn't so bad; With God's help, I think I'll fly right
     through it!

So come on blood work, and hospitals, and surgeons with skills,
and needles, and nurses, and pink ribbons, and pills.

Because from the halls of St. Vincent's to my Southside home,
I'll keep fighting each day to make sure my cancer *stays gone!*

One Thing Mama Gets to Decide

Surround yourself with only people who are
going to lift you higher.

—Oprah Winfrey

Before I had the blessing of being led to Dr. Fischer as my surgeon, I started out seeing another surgeon. She was the one who actually diagnosed me with breast cancer. After I found the lump in my breast and saw my gynecologist, she sent me for further tests at St. Vincent's Hospital. After those tests were completed, this doctor told me she would call me in a day or two with the results. Well, I waited, as patiently as I possibly could for one day. I tried my best to wait for two days, but I just couldn't. I finally called her office in the afternoon since she had not called me with any results. I got her answering service which said that her office was closed for the day. *That had to be good news*, I rationalized. If anything were wrong, she would have called right away. I waited a third day with no communication. I called her office again and left a message asking her nurse to please have the doctor call me. Nothing. That settled it. I convinced myself that nothing could possibly be wrong; if it were, she would have called by now.

On the afternoon of the fourth day after the tests, my older daughter, Claudia, had band practice. I remember it was about five in the evening because that was the time when band practice was over. I was at the practice field sitting in my car by myself waiting on Claudia to finish with band practice for the day when my cell phone rang. I looked at the number, but I didn't recognize it. I answered, "Hello."

"Is this Tonya Reid?" Someone inquired.

"Yes," I replied.

"This is Dr. Knowledge but No Wisdom (that's just what I will call her here). I am calling about your test results," she went on.

"Okay," I said, as I started to hyperventilate a little. Why, oh, why was she calling me on my cell phone at five? Surely, she wouldn't give me bad news over the phone.

"It looks like you do have breast cancer," she nonchalantly continued.

Well, then, maybe she would give me bad news over the phone. "Okay," I think I said.

"We will need to treat this aggressively. More than likely you will need to have a mastectomy," Dr. Knowledge But No Wisdom went on.

At this point, I looked up and through my tears, I saw my child walking toward my car from the band practice field. Oh dear. What was I going to do?

"Blah, blah, blah, chemotherapy, blah, blah, blah, surgery, blah, blah, my nurse will call to set you an appointment. Do you have any questions?" asked Dr. Knowledge But No Wisdom.

"No," I managed to grunt through my sobs.

"See you soon then. I am sorry about this," Dr. Knowledge But No Wisdom said as she hung up. Yeah, really sorry, I could tell.

At this point, Claudia was approaching my car, and I was sobbing my eyeballs out. I quickly wiped away my tears with the bottom of my T-shirt. Claudia was supposed to go to her dance class following band practice, so I knew if I could keep it together from Point A to Point B, that is what I needed to do. Somehow, I had managed to stop my weeping by the time she actually made it to the car. She got in and proceeded to ignore me. Sometimes having a teenager can have its advantages. I asked some cursory questions about practice, pretending to be interested while looking out my side of the car. She answered in grunts and muffled noises as she scrolled through her cell phone. I thought it was a pretty good way to avoid making eye contact. I felt sure that if I ever looked at her straight on, I would come unglued. I managed to drive her to the dance studio and drop her off for dance class without actually looking at her. She got out of the car just as I broke down. I managed to dial Tim's cell phone number and try to tell him what the doctor had just told me. It took about fifteen minutes for me to calm down enough to get the words out. He was not pleased with how the news had been delivered, to say the least, but he said all of the right things and assured me that we would get through this with God's help.

I didn't want to go home because then I would have to stay with Rachel while Tim went back to pick up

Claudia at dance (it is always tag-team-parenting). So I drove around, called my sister, and told her the news. She also said all of the right things and assured me that everything would be all right. I talked to her until it was time to pick Claudia up from the studio. I again wiped away my tears with my T-shirt bottom which now looked like I was ready to enter a wet T-shirt contest, put on a happy face, and got ready to be ignored by my teenager. Thankfully, we made it home, and she never recognized how upset I was.

Now, I am no doctor, but I certainly think that if I were delivering news like "you have cancer," I would want to bring the patient into my office and make sure he or she had a loved one with him or her when receiving the news. I really can't think of a much worse scenario than delivering this news over a cell phone when the patient is alone with no one there to offer support. Just sayin'. Some doctors, and people in general, are full of knowledge but lack the wisdom that is needed to effectively deal with certain sensitive situations. Needless to say, I did not continue with this doctor.

As mothers, we often don't get to make a lot of decisions about what we do. We get dragged along to restaurants we don't want to go to (no, we really don't want to go to McDonald's again this week), we watch TV shows we really don't want to (no, we really don't want the Disney Channel 24/7), and we participate in activities we don't particularly love (no, we actually don't adore teaching VBS as much as you think we do). We do these things because other members of our families love these things, and we want to accommodate them and want them to be happy. We love our sons, daughters, and husbands, so we go along to keep the peace. However, deciding on our own medical care and who is going to deliver it is one thing that we need to make all the decisions for ourselves. As women, we don't want to hurt feelings or cause inconveniences, but this is the one time in our lives when we can't worry about any of that, we have to put ourselves first for once and make decisions with which we are comfortable and confident. If everyone wants to keep us around for twenty, thirty, forty, or more years to continue to take care of everyone else in our families, then when we, women and mothers, are in a health crisis, we have to be able to choose the best and brightest doctors to take care of us when we need them the most. Opinions are welcomed, but the ultimate decision about what is right for us, lies with us! Let me hear an Amen! I guess it is obvious that I feel strongly about this matter.

When all of this started, I thought I would want a female surgeon since I was dealing with my female parts, after all. I thought I would feel more comfortable with a female. I quickly found out that the female I encountered was not caring and compassionate like I expected. I discovered the traits I desired in a doctor in Dr. Fischer, who happened to be male. I am sure that many people have used this female doctor and been very pleased; she just wasn't the doctor I felt comfortable with, and I happened to be the one who got to choose.

Lesson Learned: I may have to eat Chicken McNuggets three times a week, but I don't have to be treated badly by a doctor (or anyone else for that matter).

Farewell to the TATAS

Laughter is an instant vacation.

—Milton Berle

Once the date of my surgery had been set, I knew tough days lay before me. I was not looking forward to the pain, the loss, the recovery, or the unknown. I wanted to do something that would force me to dwell on happy thoughts instead of sinking into a state of depression once the deed had been done. It's not every day that a girl gets a double mastectomy after all. I thought this called for something special. I enlisted the help of my mother. She loves a good project, and she is very tech savvy. She is about the only grandmother I know who has the latest and greatest new piece of technology as soon as it hits cyberspace. We talked and came up with the idea of sending out a letter explaining what was about to happen. The letter would be accompanied by a blank card, which was to be completed by the recipient and sent back to me. We even included a return envelope that had already been stamped and addressed to me. Mom thinks of everything! I knew that this idea was a little risky and only certain people would understand by sense of humor, so I had to be selective in the people to whom I sent it. I think you will understand why. Here is the letter I sent:

Dear Friend,

The Bible tells us, "Give thanks in all circumstances, for this is God's will for you in Christ Jesus" (1 Thessalonians 5:15). Since finding out that I have breast cancer, I have struggled with how to be thankful. My doctor told me that the recurrence rate in the unaffected breast is about one percent per year after the cancer is removed from the affected breast. Since I plan to live at least sixty more years, that would be a sixty percent recurrence rate. That is not something I can accept, which has led me to my decision to say, "Farewell to the TATAS!"

Many have asked what can be done at this time to help me. Well, this is what you can do. My family and I have made the decision to go through this journey with a positive outlook, trusting God to guide us each day. I know some days will be difficult. I would like for you to take the enclosed card, and on one side, write an encouraging Bible verse, quotation, or just personal note of inspiration. On the other side of the card, please write something that will make me laugh: a joke, an embarrassing moment, a funny story, or just something that will make me smile. I look forward to receiving your card and being able to pull it out on those days when I need to be uplifted.

I hope this does not offend anyone. Believe me, I know this is a very serious situation, but I have chosen to be positive, to laugh each day, and to trust God with the future. Thank you for your prayers, and I look forward to reading what you send me.

Love,
Tonya

This letter was attached to the blank card, which my mother had made to my specifications. On the front was a picture of a very voluptuous woman with a spotlight shining on her. I figured I should go out with a bang. I also included the pre-addressed and stamped envelope. I started disseminating the letters about a week before my surgery. I probably handed out approximately twenty-five. Again, I was very selective about the people to whom I gave them because I was aware some people could just not handle this kind of thing. After I handed them out, I waited for them to start pouring in. Well, actually it was more like a trickle. I got a few before my surgery, and then after surgery, I would get two or three a week. This really worked out well because as I was recovering, I loved seeing those little envelopes when Tim brought the mail in each day. I could look forward to a good laugh when I ripped in to every one I received. And on some of those really bad, bad days, those notes were about all I could find to laugh about.

Each person who goes through a traumatic experience, like cancer, will have to decide just how he or she is going to deal with it. I felt like planning ahead for those dark days that I knew were sure to come, was a good way to prepare myself for what I was about to face. I did not want to wallow in self-pity through my entire battle with cancer, although I did spend my share of time at the punch bowl of many a pity party. These little notes allowed me to transport myself to an embarrassing moment shared with a friend or to a situation that no one but the two of us would find hilarious. Each person who sent back one of these cards made one of my days a little bit brighter. They reminded me why each of the people I chose to give the letters to is a part of my life. Sometimes you just have to laugh, so you don't cry, and these cards made me able to do that time and time again.

Lesson Learned: If you have a plan and a little help from your friends, even those horrible days can be a little more bearable.

It's a Meatloaf Kind of Day

We don't laugh because we're happy—we're happy because we laugh.

—William James

My dear husband tried his best to provide the finest possible care for me. He had been right by my side from the moment of my diagnosis on. He stayed in the hospital with me after my mastectomy, helped me change the dressing on my incisions, washed my hair when I could not raise my arms, told me I was beautiful when I most certainly was not, and kept a smile on his face all the while. I, on the other hand, have often not kept a smile on my face. Many days, my poor husband found himself encountering the *sick* wife, the *angry* wife, the *tired* wife, the *mean* wife, the *psycho* wife, or on the really bad days, the *sick-angry-tired-mean-psycho* wife. Nothing fazed him though. He steadfastly bore the brunt of any emotion or combination of emotions that I may have experienced at any moment with the utmost kindness. All women should be so blessed.

Early on, however, we did discover that he was driving me crazy by asking about 700 times a day how I was feeling. Well, I actually discovered this probably on a *mean* wife kind of day. He, of course, was just concerned and wanted to make sure that I was getting all of the proper care he could provide. I just could not take it anymore. Imagine, a husband asking so often how his wife was feeling, and if there were anything he could do for her…how rude! We had to come up with a better system. So my ever-inventive husband decided to initiate the food plan.

The food plan consisted of his asking me, "What food today?" Depending on my answer, he would know my condition (or disposition) and be prepared for how to tread. If I felt rotten, I would respond with a food that I really hated. This took a lot of thought since there are so few foods that I dislike. Usually on those days, Tim would get a response like "freeze-dried sardines" or "onion and whale blubber sandwich." Blessedly, I did not have too many horrible, horrible days. So I did not have to wrack my brain too much to come up with disgusting foods that I do not enjoy.

When Tim would ask the ever popular question, "What food today?" on the days that I felt so-so, I would respond with "meatloaf." The combination of meatloaf, mashed potatoes, butter beans, and cornbread is my favorite meal that my mother makes for me. So *meatloaf* to me means safety or everything is going to be alright, honey. That is why I used meatloaf for the average to pretty good days. It just seemed like the perfect comfort food answer.

If I was really having a great day, I would respond with "Deidra's Blueberry Cake" or "pineapple upside down cake." Of course the best days would have to be designated with sweets! Deidra's Blueberry Cake has become one of my favorite desserts since my diagnosis. My sweet friend Deidra Ledford has made several for my family (along with other food that just fades into the background when the cake is around). This cake is a multi-layer cake with blueberry filling between each layer, along with pecans and other lusciousness. It is frosted with a creamy white frosting that is scrumptious in its own right. Isn't it evident why this cake signifies a feeling extra-good day! The pineapple upside down cake is my favorite dessert that my mother makes me (it usually accompanies the meatloaf meal mentioned above.) It is my favorite dessert from childhood, and when I think about it, I start to smile. These are my two favorite desserts, so I would usually use them to describe those few and far between fantastic days.

I know this system may sound silly, and it really is. But it gave us one more way to turn a serious situation into a lighter one. Sometimes this was about all we had during the day to laugh about. On occasion, I could manage to work my way up from a "fermented salmon heads" day to a "meatloaf" day or from a "meatloaf" day to a "pineapple upside down cake" kind of day. Those days were the best. Psalm 63:5 tells us, "I will be fully satisfied as with the richest of foods; with singing lips my mouth will praise you." I know we are to praise him in all circumstances, but it was so much easier to praise him in a "Deidra's Blueberry Cake" state of mind than any other! I know when poor Tim heard on some days that it was a "meatloaf" kind of day; it just thrilled his little soul, especially after about three "onion sandwiches" in a row.

Lesson Learned: Even on those "freeze dried sardine" days, make time for a little laughter and light hearted moments.

We Are the Nu Tau Taus

A woman is like a tea bag: you cannot tell how strong she is until you put her in hot water.

—Eleanor Roosevelt

When I was in college, I pledged a sorority. Our signature color was pink, so I had been "Thinking Pink" long before my diagnosis of breast cancer. However, once the word got out that I did in fact have breast cancer, my whole world exploded with pink. Of course the pink ribbon has become the symbol of breast cancer awareness, and so people just automatically assumed that I would want to wear a pink ribbon on every single piece of clothing that I donned after my diagnosis. I never realized so many items could be found emblazoned with a pink ribbon. From hats, scarves, and jackets to socks, earrings, and underwear, I had the pink-ribboned version of them all. If people could not tell from the scarf wrapped head that I was a cancer patient, then they should certainly have been able to tell by my pink-ribboned key chain or breast cancer awareness lapel pin.

This fashion phenomenon also helped other ladies of the "Pink Ribbon Society" identify me. I quickly realized that even more than my doctors, ladies who had been through breast cancer before were the best resource for me during my journey. Doctors could tell me so much, but they couldn't help me with where to go to buy scarves or the gel that helps you keep from losing your eyelashes and eyebrows during chemotherapy treatments (which amazingly did work). Only women who had been through chemotherapy before could sympathize with me about the side effects, and only a fellow breast cancer sister could understand about how it feels when you do really lose your hair. Nobody truly understands this unless you have experienced it for yourself. I gained so much strength and inspiration from talking with women who had actually been through everything that I found myself going through. It was so nice to see them thriving after battling this awful disease fifteen years, ten years, one year, or a few months before me. Every single woman who had fought and won her battle against cancer gave me just a little bit more strength in my own battle. I would always tell myself, "If she can do it, I can do it too." They provided so much encouragement and inspiration.

God placed several key sister survivors in my path along the way. My friend Carol Harcrow was just ahead of me in her treatments, and she provided invaluable advice and encouragement. She was the first fellow traveler I met, and she helped me begin to understand how valuable the friendship and optimism from someone who has been there before can offer.

Carol was also the one who told me that once you are diagnosed with breast cancer, you are in a club where all of the members need to do all they can to support one another. That is just what she did for me. Two other "Pink Ladies" who were there to support me from the moment of my diagnosis were Ellen Hawkins and Pat Colvin. They went to my church, but it wasn't until they learned that I had breast cancer that we all really bonded. They had both been through breast cancer before me and supported me in so many ways. In fact, Ellen was the one responsible for my working through my illness.

I had asked Dr. Fischer early on how long he thought I would need to be out of work once I had my surgery. He said he thought I should plan on being out of work for approximately six to eight months since I would need chemotherapy and radiation treatments after my surgery. Hmmm…six to eight months off of work sounded like a long time, but if that is what the doctor advised, then that is what I would do. I immediately began to plan my long, leisurely mornings of sipping coffee while reading the newspaper. I would then, perhaps, enjoy diving into some of those classic novels I had been meaning to get around to reading. Later, I would certainly enjoy meditating on the meaning of life for hours on end. I could not wait to get started on all of these important endeavors. After I talked to Ellen, she told me how she was still teaching when she was taking her chemotherapy. She explained that she worked all the way through her treatments. She would work for half a day on Thursday, the day of treatment, be out on Friday, and then have the weekend to recuperate. She said by Monday, she felt well enough to be back at school teaching. She told me that working through her illness really helped her get through everything. *Well, that worked for her*, I thought, but my doctor told me to take six to eight months off. I thought I deserved six to eight months off, just to relax and regain my strength, so I made all of the arrangements with my employer to take an extended leave of absence. That lasted about two weeks. I realized that if I sat home all day, I thought about all of the "what if's." I drove myself crazy thinking about things. I couldn't even enjoy being at home by myself for thinking and worrying about things. So, I decided if Ellen could do it, then maybe I could too.

Going back to work was the best thing that I did for myself during my treatments. It got my mind off myself for the majority of the day. It got me up and out of my pajamas. It got me back on a regular schedule and that was very important for the well-being of my girls. I still had to take lots of days off to go to treatments and appointments, but at least I was not lying in bed all day just thinking of things to worry about. I will always be grateful to Ellen for just letting me know that I could continue to work if I wanted to. I also owe a big debt of gratitude to my boss, Sharon Brown, and my co-worker, Lisa Shoemaker, for doing my job as well as theirs while I was off having cancer.

Encouragement like this is so invaluable for someone going through something like breast cancer. That is why the camaraderie among its casualties is so important. Since my diagnosis, I have had the privilege of offering advice to at least three other women faced with the diagnosis. We are like members of a sorority. Since sororities and fraternities are usually identified by Greek letters, I can think of no better Greek letters for the "Sisterhood of the Pink Ribbon Society" than the Nu Tau Taus, since most of us are lucky enough to get new ta ta's at the end of our journey. It is a club you certainly don't want to become member of, but you are surely glad you have your sisters there for you when you need them.

Lesson Learned: Think pink and help a sister out at every opportunity.

How Do You Eat an Elephant?

A smile is happiness right under your nose.

—Tom Wilson

Sometimes when I stop and think about things, it is so hard for me to wrap my head around the fact that all of this was actually happening to *me*. Cancer, mastectomy, chemotherapy, oh my! Somehow I was getting through it though, one day at a time. After all, as my mother likes to remind me, "How do you eat an elephant? One bite at a time." I tried to never bite off more than I could chew when it came to this cancer thing, anyway. I am sure I will look back on this period in my life someday and think, "How did I ever do that?" I guess we do what we have to do at the time…and of course, God equips us for each season and journey in our lives. I suppose that I will look back on this period someday and marvel that I ever made it through the whole cancer thing. Mostly, I just don't think too deeply about all that was going on in my body. I chose to take the Scarlett O'Hara approach and say, "I'll think about that tomorrow."

It was funny, or maybe not funny, but I chose to view it as funny, how our family was learning to "not sweat the small stuff" through this whole process. Again, not biting off more than we could chew, as we have been known to do in the past. Things that would once have sent me over the edge, now didn't even register as a blip on my radar. For example, early in December, Claudia was scheduled to march in the local Christmas parade with the high school band. I had missed most all of her performances during football season due to chemotherapy. Now that I was feeling better, I was determined to see the parade. It didn't matter what the temperature or how many germ-infested onlookers I had to endure. Luckily, my good friend Gina Turner, made arrangements for Tim, Rachel, and me, to join her in viewing the parade from the comfort of a beautiful building in historic downtown Gadsden. We had the luxury of being able to be watch the parade from the second story of this cozy, warm office building with a great view from its bank of picture windows. We all settled in to watch the parade as we anxiously awaited the arrival of the Southside High School Band to appear. It just so happened that our band was toward the end of the parade, so we got to see lots of beauty queens, clown cars, horses, Santa Clauses, and baby Jesuses while we waited. Apparently, Rachel wanted to get a little more comfortable during the long procession, so she removed her tennis shoes to settle in for the duration. Suddenly, a not-so-pleasant odor began emanating through the air. We quickly discovered that the source of the foul stench was Rachel's stinky socks. Do you want to know what her response to this discovery was? "Well, I have been wearing them for four days in a row." Now, B.C. (before cancer) this would have sent me into a royal tizzy! I would have lectured Rachel, lectured Tim, been angry at myself, yelled at Claudia just because, and probably made us all miserable for the next week by making sure Rachel had on spotless, clean, fresh-smelling socks each day. Want to know what my reaction was on that particular Monday night? I told Rachel to point her feet away from me, so I didn't have to smell them.

By this point, I was just proud that my girls were making it to school dressed, fed, and with homework (mostly) completed. And if dressed consisted of recycled socks on some days, so be it. I was not going to worry about it. God's word tells us in Matthew 6:28–30, "And why do you worry about clothes? See how the flowers of the field grow. They do not labor or spin. Yet I tell you that not even Solomon in all his splendor was dressed like one of these. If that is how God clothes the grass of the field, which is here today and tomorrow is thrown into the fire, will he not much more clothe you—you of little faith?" Whew! Thank you, Lord, for one less thing for me to have to worry about!

Lesson Learned: Clean socks are overrated; concentrate on the things that really matter.

In Brenda Ladun's Shadow

Life's most urgent question is: What are you
doing for others?

—Martin Luther King, Jr.

I am not sure just how far-reaching Brenda Ladun's
influence extends, but she is a beloved newscaster in
my little corner of the world. She expertly delivers the
news to viewers around my area each day at 6:00 p.m.
and 10:00 p.m. on ABC 33/40. Besides being beautiful,
articulate, and trustworthy, Brenda is also a two time
breast cancer survivor. Yes, two time. Both times that
Brenda Ladun suffered through cancer, she remained
on the air and was very candid and open about her
health. If viewers didn't love Brenda Ladun before her
cancer, they certainly fell head over heels for her while
watching as she gracefully met all of the challenges that
came along with the illness while maintaining her poise
each day on air with countless people watching. Brenda
has also written two books about dealing with cancer:
*Getting Better, Not Bitter: A Spiritual Prescription for
Breast Cancer* and *Behind the Scenes of Breast Cancer: A*

News Anchor Tells Her Story of Body and Soul Recovery. She may not technically be America's sweetheart, but she is most definitely Northeast Alabama's sweetheart, and she would be America's sweetheart if ABC 33/40 had a signal strong enough, believe me. Everyone loves Brenda.

This fact became quite evident shortly after my journey started. Once you are diagnosed with cancer (especially of the breast variety and especially in Alabama), everybody wants to tell you all about Brenda Ladun. Somehow people know about everything she did, who she used, how it turned out, and how they would feel so much better if you used the same doctors as she did. Apparently, everyone has read both of her books from cover to cover and watched her every single day on the news as she bravely triumphed over the horrible disease. I started receiving copies of her books almost immediately. People would give books to me at church, send them to me in the mail, and drop them off to me at home. I probably ended up with about six copies of one and four or five of the other. I tried to tell people that I had already read them, but they insisted that I had probably read the other one (not the one they were giving me), and gave me a copy anyway, just in case I needed it. Of course, I did read both books and found them very uplifting and helpful.

After reading one of Brenda's books, I discovered that we did indeed share some of the same healthcare providers. This fact did seem to send a huge sigh of relief through the many people worried about me. I was so glad I could do something to relieve some of their fears. I am really surprised that any other doctors who are located in the Birmingham area and deal with breast cancer have any patients whatsoever since Brenda named names in her books because I can tell you from personal experience, people think only the doctors Brenda used are worth any salt. Yes, she is that beloved.

After I kept getting more and more copies of the book, I decided I would try to contact Brenda and let her know how much I enjoyed the books and what an impact they continued to have on those dealing with breast cancer. I looked her up on the ABC/33 website and found her e-mail address. I quickly composed an email telling her about my situation and explaining how her books had been so helpful to me (all 287 copies). I sent the note and thought that maybe one day an assistant may run across it and let Brenda see it, and she might smile. I assumed she got hundreds of e-mails like this, considering the prevalence of breast cancer. Well, just imagine my surprise when I checked my e-mail the very next day and spotted a reply from Mrs. Ladun herself! She had written back a personal note of encouragement to me, and not only that, she had given me her personal cell phone number in case I needed to call her to talk! It was a short note, but nonetheless, a personal reply. No wonder people love this woman. She took the time out of her busy schedule to respond to a woman she did not know who was going through a crisis. And giving me her personal cell phone number...wow! I avoid giving my cell phone number to certain family members for fear they will drive me nuts. She has more courage than I have, and talk about living out her faith, my goodness. She ministered more to me in that short little e-mail than she could have ever imagined, I am sure. She showed me that even though she had long beaten cancer herself, she still cared about those who were fighting it now. Her note energized me! It made me think, *If Brenda can beat cancer, I can too*. I never used that cell phone number, but I have no doubt that if I called Brenda up on one of those really bad days (like a chicken gizzard and mustard pie kind of day), she would have talked me right through it.

Her actions made me want to be a "Brenda" for someone. Of course I don't come with the celebrity and name recognition of the Ladun variety, but she made me realize what a little encouragement can do for someone. Brenda Ladun is not the only breast cancer survivor who has provided much needed cheering on for me. The majority of it has come from regular gals like me who just happened to find themselves battling this awful disease too, and their kind words and phone calls have meant just as much as Brenda's sentiments. They have prayed for me, sent cards to me, and called to check on me. They have all taught me that I need to pay it forward, and be that kind of encouraging presence in the life of the next woman who finds herself in the awful position of having to hear the words, "You have breast cancer." Yes, I have been there, and because of that, maybe, just maybe, I can help someone else get through those hard, hard days she will be sure to face. After all, if Brenda (and Tonya) can do it, so can she!

Lesson Learned: Never underestimate the power of a little encouragement.

Dear Cancer

Dear Cancer,

I just wanted to take this opportunity to let you know exactly how I feel about you. You came into my life so suddenly. Certainly, at forty-two years of age, your appearance was not something that I was looking for. However, what an appearance you made! Bursting onto the scene when I was least expecting you! Things were rolling along pretty smoothly in my life, and then here you come and turn my whole world upside down. Like a jealous boyfriend, you slowly began dominating all of my time and attention. I couldn't think about anything else but you. Everything in my entire existence slowly started revolving around you. I would wake up thinking about you, make every decision with you in mind, and go to bed worrying about what you were going to do to me. Would I be one of the unfortunate who would succumb to your destruction by letting you run my life and take me down by sucking all of the life blood out of me? Or would I be one of the lucky ones who would catch you early and refuse to let you control me?

Let's be honest, I let you run the show for awhile there. I was so scared and confused. I couldn't quite wrap my head around what was happening to me. Decisions had to be made so quickly. All anyone ever wanted to talk about was you…cancer this, cancer that. It was like you took my identity away from me. No one could talk to me anymore without talking about you! I hated that. When did my life start depending on you? Finally, I realized, it didn't.

Yes, you did take many things away from me. I'll start with the two biggest (well, okay, they were never that big). But you did take my body. It will never be the same because of you. I hate you for that. You took time away from my family. I missed out on so many things because of you. I missed seeing Claudia march in most of her football games this season. I can never get that back and will forever regret that I did not get to experience such an important part of her school experience. I missed Halloween and trunk-or-treat with Rachel. I know that sounds silly, but she is eight years old, and I know that I won't have many more opportunities to get to do that with her. We always have so much fun going to the church and walking around with friends to all of the cars and filling up her trick-or-treat bag. I will never forgive you for those memories you took away from me. I missed out on so much of my life during those months that you were with me. But like a bad boyfriend, I have now gotten rid of you.

I have now finished my sixth and last chemotherapy treatment. I now bid you adieu, prayerfully forever. I wish to no longer have any association of any sort with you. You have really hurt my reputation. Though you did manage to take many things from me in our short but significant time together, there are some things that you gave me while we were together that I must thank you for. You gave me a greater appreciation for my relationship with my Heavenly Father. I know that he is with me each and every day and that when you were too much for me to handle, you were no match for him. You gave me a greater appreciation for my family. I hate that they had to be associated with you because of me, but their strength and love in the face of adversity has been truly inspiring. You gave me a greater appreciation for my friends. It still amazes me to think about some of the things that have been done on my behalf during the course of this journey. My family has been cooked for, cleaned up after, prayed for, shopped for, and taxied around just to get the list started. Once I realized that I was not going to allow you to overpower me, you gave me a sense of humor about it all. It is true that some days you just have to laugh, so you don't cry, but I found out early on that I just felt so much better if I laughed instead of cried. So, I really have tried to laugh my way through it, tears streaming down my face and all, which brings us to the end of this portion of our journey together. Yes, I know I still have to face some more treatments and probably scans, check-ups, and probes forever, but I say the worst is over!

Chemotherapy is now behind me! It certainly could have been worse, and I thank God that I was able to handle the treatments as well as I did. I think it is nothing short of miraculous. Thank you, Lord, for Phenergan, saltines, and Tonya Noodle Soup. Thank you for good friends who pray and take care of my family. Thank you that my family has handled this portion of the journey so well and in such good spirits. Thank you for being bigger than cancer and never, ever leaving me alone in the fight!

Sincerely,
Tonya

And the Special Treatment Ends

> In three words, I can sum up everything I've
> learned about life: it goes on.
>
> —Robert Frost

When you are dealing with cancer, you feel almost as if you are living in a sort of parallel world. You are going through the motions of your everyday life, but you are also dealing with all of the cancer issues as well. When I was taking my radiation treatments, I would work all day, go to radiation in the afternoons, be a soccer mom after I picked up the girls (even though I was hauling to dance and gymnastics and not soccer), and then when we finally made it home, my family had the nerve to want food and clean underwear. It was really bizarre. A lot of the tasks that my girls had depended on me to do B.C. (before cancer) they now had to depend on their dad to do, or they actually had to do them for themselves (horror of horrors). Imagine, an eighth grader discovering she could actually pack her own lunch for school! We all just had to learn how to live with the diagnosis of cancer, and all that it entailed.

I had learned to live with fat thighs and my inability to keep my refrigerator organized years ago, so I could figure out how to live with a cancer diagnosis too. I just hated that my entire family had to do the same, but they never complained. They were with me every step of the way, and they pitched in to do anything I needed them to do. And we made it! Hallelujah! Praise the Lord!

After living through the cancer diagnosis, the chemotherapy treatments, the hair loss, and the radiation treatments, Tim, Claudia, Rachel, and I could hardly wait for things to get back to normal. We just forgot exactly what "normal" was for our family. The end of all of my treatments and doctors' visits pretty much coincided with the end of the school year. Two events occurred that, to me, signified that the Reids had returned to the land of the ordinary, and all of the special treatment, good or bad, had come to an end. The bubble I had been living in had finally burst. The first event was Claudia's eighth grade graduation.

Amazingly enough, even with all that had gone on throughout the school year, Claudia had somehow managed to run for and be elected president of the student government association for her school. During the school year, the SGA traveled to the state convention held in Birmingham, and Claudia competed in the speech competition there. Cancer even followed us to the SGA convention though. Tim, Rachel, and I travelled to Birmingham on the day of the competition to listen to all of the contestants deliver their speeches. We anxiously awaited the results once the students had finished speaking. We were all so proud when Claudia tied for first alternate in the state! The winner and the two students who tied for first alternate were then invited to deliver their speeches at the luncheon for all of the attendees at the convention. Well guess what? I had a doctor's appointment I had to get to. We waited as long as we possibly could, but we had to leave before Claudia got to present her speech in front of the entire gathering. Cancer struck once again.

At the end of the school year, Claudia's SGA sponsor, Sherry Johnson, and the administrators of the school, asked her to deliver the speech again at the eighth grade graduation ceremony. She was beyond excited! She practiced and practiced and even added some additional remarks at the end of the speech addressed directly to her classmates. All we talked about around our house for weeks was the upcoming graduation ceremony and the speech. The day of the graduation finally rolled around, and it was typical chaos around our house, as usual. Rachel had a field trip scheduled for that day, and after much debate, Tim and I had decided that she could go ahead and go on the field trip. She had missed so much fun stuff throughout the year that we hated to have her miss her end of the year field trip too. It was decided that Tim would take Rachel to her school and drop her off for the field trip and then meet me at Claudia's graduation ceremony. As he was running out the door, we realized that we had no batteries for the video camera, so he would also swing by the store to pick up batteries before coming to the graduation. We are always so prepared.

Claudia and I drove to the church where her graduation was taking place. She got settled with her classmates, and I found great seats on the second row of pews for Tim and me. It was the perfect spot for enjoying my precious baby presenting her speech and for Tim to capture the entire event on video. I waited for his arrival, and I waited, and I waited. I kept looking at my watch, and I soon began to worry if he was going to arrive in time. Rachel's school was right down the road from the church and so was the Dollar General where he would have stopped for batteries. Finally, I sent him a text, "Where are you?"

He responded, "Leaving the store." Great! He should be arriving at the church in just a few minutes. Well, he didn't.

I sent another text, "Are you almost here?"

He responded, "Parking the car." Whew! I was so glad. Graduation was going to begin in about ten minutes. I was really beginning to get antsy.

I felt my phone vibrate. I looked down and saw that I had a text message from Tim, "Is it in the gym?" No, No, No, he could not be asking me that!

My fingers started going crazy as I began texting more quickly than a preteen girl, "It is at Southside Baptist Church not at the school!"

He replied, "On the way."

Now Claudia's school is not hundreds of miles away from Southside Baptist Church, but that is what it felt like as I waited for Tim to drive from Rainbow Middle School to the church. The time for graduation to begin arrived, and Tim was still not there. The principal got up to make her opening remarks, and Tim was still not there. Just as Claudia stood up to make her way to the podium, Tim slid into the seat next to me on the pew. Thank you, Lord! We didn't even have time to have a whispered exchange about how this miscommunication could possibly have happened before our older daughter was standing at the microphone delivering her speech in front of the audience. She was flawless. She spoke about learning about climbing mountains throughout the past year and taking life one step at a time. Many in the audience, I am sure, thought she was referring to typical middle school mumbo jumbo, but we, she, Tim, and I, understood those words held a much deeper meaning. That speech was just one more reminder of how cancer had affected my family. My daughter had not come out unscathed by any means, but more mature, more caring, and a little less innocent about what life will throw at you when you least expect it.

The second event that signified I could now be viewed as a regular citizen and not Tonya-the-lady-with-breast-cancer occurred when school let out for summer. By that time, enough hair had grown back on my head to make a private first class jealous. I had promised Rachel that I would continue to wear my scarves until school was over. She was still very sensitive about the whole hair issue. She absolutely did not want me showing up at her school looking like Mr. Clean. However, now that I did have enough hair to actually cover my head plus the fact that it was getting to be summertime in Alabama, I was ready to shed the scarves for good. The first time I went out in public with no scarf on my head was the first Saturday after school was out. As usual, the girls and I had to be in several different places in a short amount of time. I had to drop Claudia off at dress rehearsal for her upcoming dance recital. I then had to run Rachel over to a birthday party. Tim was going to meet Rachel at the party after he got off work to pick her up there. I was then to go back to pick Claudia up at dress rehearsal and help her with any last minute preparations she needed. I succeeded in dropping off Claudia at her practice. I must admit I felt a little self-conscious about being without a scarf. I had worn one for so long that I felt a little off-balance without one. Rachel and I were on our way to the birthday party. I took a wrong turn and had to backtrack. This of course put us behind schedule. I was rushing to get her to the location on time. Rushing a bit too much apparently, because next thing I knew, I saw flashing lights behind me. Yep, I was being pulled over.

The police officer approached my window and asked if I realized I was speeding. I told him I was sorry and handed him my license and insurance card. He walked back to his car to do whatever it is they do back there. Now imagine how I looked, practically bald headed, save the whisper-thin layer of dark fuzz covering the majority of my head. Mr. Policeman saw this picture and compared it to my driver's license picture, which showed me with my helmet hair which I sported B.C. (before cancer). Surely, he could not think the lack of hair was a fashion statement. I was well-over the age to do such a thing. I thought he would probably issue me a warning because it was obvious I was just getting over some terrible disease. He would not think of giving me a ticket. I wasn't going that fast. I watched as Mr. Policeman slowly walked back to my car. I prepared myself to be gracious as he issued a warning to slow it down and asked about what horrible malady I was experiencing, but instead, he handed me back my license, my insurance card, and a speeding ticket. He didn't even question the whole hair thing. Of course, my license also said I weighed one-hundred and ten pounds, and he didn't question that either.

I didn't know if I wanted to slap him or hug him. Slap him for giving me the ticket, of course. It didn't matter that I actually was speeding. But then, I also wanted to hug him because he was the first person in a long time to look at me for me and not look at me as the lady who had breast cancer. I don't know if it would have made a bit of difference if I had mentioned my ordeal of the past year to him or that this was my first day out in public with nothing covering my head and that I felt a little off kilter. I could have tried crying and using the sympathy card, but I didn't. I was just a law-breaker, and he was just Mr. Policeman. He did his job, and I took my ticket. Many people asked afterward why I didn't tell him about the cancer, or why I didn't cry. I guess because I was just so ready to be "normal" again, and "normal" people get speeding tickets. Normal people forget to buy batteries for the camera for special occasions. Normal people forget to tell their husbands important details sometimes. Normal people run late, have messy houses, lose things, eat cereal for supper, and forget to send lunch money for their children.

I had spent a year only thinking about cancer. I was ready to think about the day to day normal activities that I missed so much. I was actually a little excited to get the ticket, because I thought maybe, just maybe, Mr. Policeman looked at me and saw a lady who was speeding and never even thought about cancer at all. This was the day I had waited for. Thank you, God, for my speeding ticket!

Lesson Learned: Even a speeding ticket can be a blessing in disguise. Thank you, Lord, for every blessing!